TABLE OF CONTENTS

Chapter 1.	**Enhancing your Reiki Practice with Reikiatsu**	1
	What exactly is Reikiatsu?	1
	So What is the Meridian System?	1
	What is Ki?	2
	What is Yin and Yang?	3
	Kyo and Jitsu	3
	Circulating and Directing Ki	4
	1) Maintaining a correct posture	4
	2) Breathing from the Hara	5
	3) Meditating from your centre	6
	4) The Microcosmic Orbit	7
	Circulating Ki through the Chakras	10
	5) The Macrocosmic Orbit	12
Chapter 2.	**The Meridian System**	14
	The Stomach Meridian	18
	The Spleen Meridian	20
	The Heart Meridian	22
	The Small Intestine Meridian	24
	The Bladder Meridian	26
	The Kidney Meridian	28
	The Pericardium Meridian	30
	The Triple Heater Meridian	32
	The Gall Bladder Meridian	34
	The Liver Meridian	36
	The Lung Meridian	38
	The Large Intestine Meridian	40
	The Governing Vessel	42
	The Conception Vessel	44
Chapter 3.	**The Five Elements**	46
	The Wood Meridians	47
	The Fire Meridians	48
	The Earth Meridians	48
	The Metal Meridians	49
	The Water Meridians	49

Chapter 4.	**Reikiatsu Sessions**	50
	Directing Ki into the meridians	50
	Letting your intuition guide you	50
	Hand Positions	51
	No Contact Technique	51
	Two Thumb Technique	52
	Two Finger Technique	52
	Gentle Touch Technique	53
	Grip Technique	53
	Earth Element Sessions	54
	The Stomach Meridian Reikiatsu Session	55
	The Spleen Meridian Reikiatsu Session	57
	Metal Element Sessions	59
	The Lung Meridian	59
	The Large Intestine Meridian	61
	Water Element Sessions	63
	The Bladder Meridian	63
	The Kidney Meridian	66
	Wood Element Sessions	68
	The Gall Bladder Meridian	68
	The Liver Meridian	70
	Fire Element Sessions	72
	The Heart Meridian	73
	The Small Intestine Meridian	74
	The Pericardium Meridian	76
	The Triple Heater Meridian	77
	The Three Treasures	79
	Merging Rivers Sessions	80
	The Governing Vessel	80
	The Conception Vessel	83

Reikiatsu

THE REIKI PRACTITIONER'S GUIDE TO WORKING WITH THE MERIDIANS

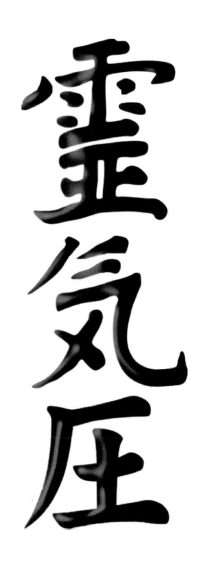

PAUL N. BESHARA

Copyright © 2017 Paul N. Beshara

All rights reserved.

The procedures and techniques contained in this book regarding health and well-being are based on the training, research, as well as, the personal and professional experiences of the author. As each person is unique and each situation is individual, if there arises any question regarding the effects or procedure of any Reikiatsu session, the author advises that the practitioner has their client check with a qualified health professional.

Cover Design: Paul Beshara

Illustrations: Paul Beshara

Cover Photo Credits:
- Lotus pose [ostill] © 123RF.com
- Hands on vortex [Nicola Zalewski] © 123RF.com

Interior Photo Credits:
- Lying down pose - [Aleksandr Davydov] © 123RF.com - Page 4
- Seiza pose - [Aleksandr Davydov] © 123RF.com - Pages 4, & 7
- Seiza pose - [Aleksandr Davydov] © 123RF.com - Pages 5, 8, & 9
- Lotus pose [ostill] © 123RF.com - Page 19
- Sunset Tai Chi - [Oleksandr Mudretsov] © 123RF.com - Page 12
- Reiki session - [Wavebreak Media Ltd] © 123RF.com - Page 51
- Two finger technique - [Branislav Ostojic] © 123RF.com - Page 52
- Two thumb technique - [Branislav Ostojic] © 123RF.com - Page 52
- Gentle touch technique - [Branislav Ostojic] © 123RF.com - Page 53
- Grip technique - [Branislav Ostojic] © 123RF.com - Page 53
- All other images reproduced through Creative Commons

All rights reserved. No part of this publication may be reproduced, distributed, or transmitted in any form or by any means, including photocopying, recording, or other electronic or mechanical methods, without the prior written permission of the author, except in the case of brief quotations embodied in critical reviews and certain other noncommercial uses permitted by copyright law.

ACKNOWLEDGEMENTS

I wish to express heartfelt gratitude to all my guides and teachers. In particular, I wish to acknowledge Reiki Master, Gail Rose, who awakened me to a whole other world and taught me my First and Second Degree Reiki in 1993. Special mention also has to be given to Jan Vincent of Blue Crane Studio, who taught me the Meridian System and Shiatsu in 1995. I also want to thank Reiki Master, Roberta Della-Picca, who taught and initiated me as a Reiki Master in 1998.

It would be impossible to fully express how thankful I am, that the spirit of Mikao Usui lives on through Reiki and the timeless teachings of Usui Shiki Ryoho.

It would be also impossible, to individually thank all of my clients and friends that have been an invaluable part of this learning process, but I hold you forever in my heart.

These wonderful teachers all contributed to the evolving process of this book and it is through their shared knowledge that I first envisioned and am now content with the final result.

Reiki Blessings of Love & Light

DEDICATION

With sincere gratitude and appreciation, to my loving partner, Debra, who always supports my every endeavour, and to my wonderful children, Rebecca, Crystal, Alex, Amber, and Coral, who love me unconditionally, I dedicate this book.

Chapter 5   **Specific Point - Reikiatsu Sessions**   85

    Stomach 36 - 3 Mile Point - Releasing worry   85
    Stomach 25 - Heaven's Pivot - Restoring calmness   85
    Spleen 4 - Grandfather Grandson - Restoring self-confidence   86
    Spleen 6 - Three Yin Intersection - Freedom from toxic emotions   86
    Bladder 52 - Will Chamber - Uplifting the spirit   86
    Gallbladder 21 - Shoulder Well - Expressing emotions   87
    Gallbladder 34 - Yang Mound Spring - Inner peace   87
    Gallbladder 44 - Yin Portals of the Foot - Resolution of anger   87
    Liver 1 - Great Esteem- Increasing self-esteem   88
    Liver 2 - Moving Between - Expressing emotions in a healthy way   88
    Liver 3 - Great Rushing - Embracing serenity   88
    Lung 1- Central Treasury - Letting go of grief   89
    Pericardium 6 - Inner Gate - Calming the flames   89
    Pericardium 7 - Great Mount - Protecting the heart   89
    Triple Heater 5 - Outer Frontier Gate - Overcoming insecurities   90
    Triple Heater 7 - Wind Screen - Becoming care-free   90
    Kidney 3 - Supreme Stream - Fearless empowerment   90
    Kidney 6 - Shining Sea - Flowing with grace and ease   91
    Large Intestine 4 - Union Valley - Inspired living   91
    Large Intestine 11 - Crooked Pond - Freeing the prisoner   91
    Small Intestine 5 - Yang Valley- Experiencing self-determination   92
    Small Intestine 19 - Palace of Hearing - Listening to your heart   92

    Conclusion   93
    About the author   94

FOREWARD

From the time I first began to practice Reiki, in 1993, I felt that the traditional Reiki hand positions were only the beginning. Once introduced to Reiki, I became open to the unlimited possibilities of actively participating in the flow of Universal Life Force energy. I fully embraced this subtle, yet powerful, energy which was able to balance the energies of human and other life forms. I loved how it facilitated a more harmonious flow of life force energy throughout their systems.

It is true, that the traditional hand positions of Reiki do happen to cover the principle Chakra positions and some of the meridians and their points. Upon studying Shiatsu, however, I found that my Reiki practice, as well as my own well being, was enhanced by a greater understanding of the Meridian System and its relationship to health and vitality. This ancient wisdom led me to an acceleration in my spiritual evolution.

Applying Reiki, with intention, directly on the meridians, maximizes the flow of Ki through the channels and removes blockages that are obstacles to the well-being of body and soul.

There is a wealth of knowledge out there that addresses Acupressure, Acupuncture, Shiatsu, and the Meridian System. However, I have not seen any that specifically assists Reiki practitioners to gain a greater understanding of the meridians and how it applies to their Reiki practice. This void appeared to me as an opportunity to share my understanding of the Meridian System with other Reiki Practitioners and Masters, such as yourself.

I have endeavoured to make this book as user-friendly as possible so that it brings you a greater energetic understanding of yourself and those you serve.

There are two ways that you can use this book. Both are offered to you as tools to enhance your Reiki with Reikiatsu:

1. You can choose to simply bypass Chapter 1 and begin with your current understanding of Reiki and apply it to the Meridian System as it is explained in Chapter 2 and beyond.

or

2. You can begin your study with Chapter 1, which offers powerful techniques for increasing and directing the flow of Universal Life Force Energy, known to you as Reiki. By practicing the exercises in this chapter, you will learn to consciously direct, and amplify, the flow of Reiki throughout your own Meridian System. With this experience, your ability to transport Reiki, and bring balance and harmony to the meridians will become highly advanced.

Much Light, Love, and Reiki blessings,

Paul Beshara.

CHAPTER 1

ENHANCING YOUR REIKI PRACTICE WITH REIKIATSU

WHAT EXACTLY IS REIKIATSU?

Reikiatsu is an advanced Reiki modality that accesses the infinite flow of Universal Life Force Energy (The "Ki" in Reiki) and directs it to flow through you to the channels and points of the Meridian System. By applying gentle pressure on these traditional acupressure points, or simply resting your hands on specific meridians, the flow of Reiki brings balances their energy flow and disperses obstacles to wellness. For you, as a Reiki practitioner, to awaken to the power of Reikiatsu you will require a basic understanding of the meridians, their points, and their general functions.

In Chapter 1, we will first go over the basics of the terms and principles of the Meridian System and some energetic practices, which will amplify the flow of Universal Life Force Energy within and through you. We will study the meridians in more depth in the later chapters. The scope of this book is to provide you with a working knowledge of Reikiatsu so that your practice of Reiki will be greatly enhanced.

Some of this material may be familiar to you, and some of it may be entirely new.

Don't worry about trying to absorb everything all at once. The new always becomes familiar as we get used to it. Approach this book with an open mind and you will be greatly rewarded.

SO WHAT IS THE MERIDIAN SYSTEM?

As a Reiki Practitioner, and as a living soul, whether you presently understand anything about the meridians or the Meridian System, you are wholly engaged in this energetic dance by your very existence. You already know that the Universe is comprised of Infinite Cosmic Energy vibrating at different frequencies. The frequency at which this Cosmic Energy vibrates determines how it shows up and is experienced, by all of life.

The Meridian System is a enlightened understanding of the way in which this cosmic energy flows throughout the human body. The Meridian System maps these energy pathways as they travel though, and access all parts of the body. These pathways or channels are an energetic distribution network that supplies the body with vital fundamental substances such as blood, bodily fluids, and Ki.

These essences are the foundation of life and health. When there is an imbalance or blockage in the flow of these substances, a person's vitality and emotional well-being are impaired.

WHAT IS KI?

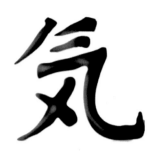

*"Conceived of as having no name,
it is the Originator of heaven and earth;
Conceived of as having a name, it is the Mother of all Things."*
~ *Tao Te Ching*

To understand and work with the Meridian System, as a Reiki practitioner, we must begin with the basic principles that are its foundation. The first is an understanding of Ki as the essence of the Absolute Universe.

Sometime between 3000 and 2000 B.C., the Chinese came to understand the existence of a vital life force energy which they called Chi. They determined that all matter, animate and inanimate, is composed of and infused with this universal energy. This was not a new idea. Many of the ancient cultures understood this life force energy as the Breath of Life or Spirit. What was new, however, was that the Chinese developed and documented a system that followed the flow of Chi through the human body. They also postulated that along these channels were specific points that could be accessed with acupressure, or acupuncture, to facilitate the removal of energy blockages within a living body. These cardinal points, they associated with various organs or bodily functions. They discovered that when energy was intentionally channelled into these meridians by way of a needle or simply touch, these points responded by allowing the Chi energy to flow and balance the system.

For the purpose of this book, since you are already familiar with the name of this Chi energy as Ki, (the Japanese word for Chi) this is the term we will use. Ki is the Universal Life Force Energy that flows in Rei-ki.

So what exactly is the Ki in Reiki?

If you were to meditate on anything in the Universe and contemplate on its origin, you would always find that it appears to have mysteriously arisen out of something else. When you follow the origin of that "something else" back to its beginning, you find it, too, originated from something else. When you follow everything back to its original source, it appears to have arisen out of nearly nothing.

This Original Source is beyond identification. It is transcends being called anything and yet everything has arisen from it. Some people have called this source Spirit. Others called it by countless other names. The Chinese called it Chi. The Greeks called it Pneuma. The Hebrews called it Ruach. In India, they called it Prana. The Japanese refer to it as Ki. These are the names we have ascribed to the un-nameable, indivisible Source Energy that is the origin of all substance and life in the Universe.

This original Ki is that Non-being from which all Being-ness sprung. It is what you were before you were born, and is you now. This Ki, that you are now and always were, is the same Ki that is also the Sun, both now, and before it existed. Ki is the unifying factor in all that is. We are all that One and it is out of that Oneness that we, individually, make our appearance.

WHAT IS YIN AND YANG?

All that springs out of Oneness is universally experienced as Duality and Opposition. This is expressed through the principle of Yin and Yang.

"Always without desire we must be found, if its deep mystery we would sound;
But if desire always within us be, its outer fringe is all that we shall see.
Under these two aspects, it is really the same;
but as development takes place, it receives the different names.
Together we call them the Mystery.
Where the Mystery is the deepest, is the gate of all that is subtle and wonderful."
~ Tao Te Ching

The concept of Yin and Yang originated in China about the same time as the Meridian System. This principle maintains that the Absolute Universe is One Life Force, and it is with the appearance of two opposing forces that the relative world is born. All things that come into existence, through and from the One, appear as inseparable and contradictory opposites. Some examples of this would be Masculine (Yang) / Feminine (Yin), and Darkness (Yin) / Light (Yang). These two opposites attract and complement each other and as the Yin/Yang symbol depicts, each of the forces always contains an element of the other aspect, within its core.

KYO AND JITSU

We now must come to an understanding about balance and imbalance, within living systems. When the yin and yang aspects of Ki are balanced, the living system is in a state of vitality. When the yin and yang become unbalanced, the living system displays a dis-eased state. Excessive yang results in over-active organic activity. When yin energy is predominate, organic activity is under-active. In both cases, the imbalance results in impaired health and leads to illness.

This principle applies to all of creation. You may have noticed when walking along a river bank, that wherever the water does not flow freely, that is where the garbage gathers. We call this stagnation. It is the same within our bodily systems. Just as we require blood to flow freely through our circulatory system to remain healthy, we also need Ki to flow freely through our Meridian System. When blood does not flow freely, inharmonious conditions occur, and illness is the outcome. The same thing may be said about the Meridian System. When Ki energy does not flow freely through the meridians, an imbalance occurs. This results in points along the meridians that have an excess of energy, and points that are depleted in energy. The points that have an excess of energy, are called Jitsu, and the points that are depleted, are called Kyo. By moving energy from Jitsu (high concentration) areas to Kyo (low concentration) locations, balance is restored.

Like the ancient art of acupuncture, acupressure, and meridian massage, Reikiatsu focuses on restoring the Yin/Yang energy balance and bringing harmony to Ki of the body.

CIRCULATING AND DIRECTING KI

As a Reiki practitioner, you are already accustomed to being a clear channel of Light Energy known as Rei-Ki. Through your connection with the Infinite Storehouse of Universal Life Force, energy flows through you lovingly, and naturally. To begin working with the meridians and practicing Reikiatsu, you will be exercising what is known as Circulating and Directing Ki. This practice directs the flow of Ki both within and beyond you. When this flow is intentionally directed through a meridian, or meridian point, it can restore the balance of yin and yang.

By practicing the following six principles, you will become proficient in enhancing, directing the flow of Ki, and balancing the yin/yang energies of the meridian system:

1) Maintaining a correct posture.

2) Breathing from the Hara.

3) Meditating from your centre.

4) Consciously Circulating Ki - The Microcosmic Orbit

5) Consciously Directing Ki - The Macrocosmic Orbit

6) Transporting Ki

1) Maintaining a correct Posture - If you are going to channel Ki clearly and freely, your mind and body must not hinder its flow. This free flow of energy can only be achieved with a calm mind and correct posture. The natural state of your body is calmness. Holding tension within your body causes it to fall out of its natural state. The good thing is, your body already knows how to correct itself. Calmness returns when you release any tension you are holding. This can happen through establishing correct posture. It is from a state of serenity, that the highest and clearest parts of your consciousness are able to direct the flow of Ki.

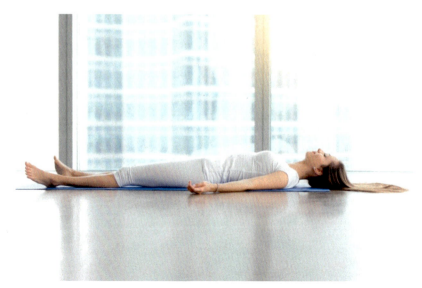

One easy way to learn this tension release is to lie flat on your back, on the floor, or on your Reiki table, and simply relax. Don't try to adjust your posture with commands. That will only cause more tension. Rather, pay attention to any tension you may feel and allow it to relax. Start with the top of your head and journey on down. You may notice tension in your jaw… Let it relax. Breathe light into the area of tension, and relax. Continue on down throughout your whole body. After you are totally relaxed, pay close attention to how you feel. This centred calmness is how you should feel, at all times, in any posture. Totally calm and relaxed.

Now try to repeat this exercise sitting, as well as standing up. Begin with the top of your head, and work your way down, releasing any tension you are holding. It would be good, to practice both of these positions until you know what it "feels" like, to be totally at peace, and without tension, or stress. *This calm serene state, is what we mean when we say, "Having correct posture".*

2) Breathing from the Hara - Breathing is essential, to life as you know it. The word Ki, we have previously mentioned, is the same as Pneuma, which is the Greek word for "Breath", and means, " the vital spirit, soul, or creative force of a person".

When you inhale, you receive this vitality, and when you exhale, you give it.
This is the yin and yang, of the rhythm of life.

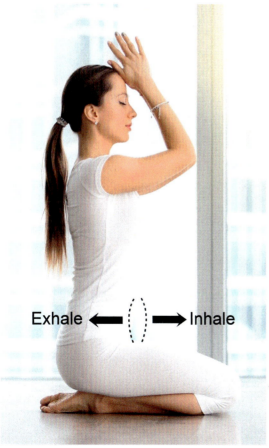

To learn to access and direct Ki goes, hand in hand, with learning how to breathe correctly.

Breathing, you already know how to do. Breathing correctly, on the other hand, is something that most people have to learn. A breath that is to stimulate, and extend the flow of Ki, must take place deep down in your body. This is called breathing from your diaphragm, or belly. We will call it, "*Breathing from the Hara*", the Japanese word for this area.

Most people breathe only into their chest. This is very shallow breathing. Shallow breathing is short rapid breaths. Shallow breathing always accompanies anxiety.

If you are anxious, you breathe in short gasps. If you breathe shallow, you become anxious.

This is because when you shallow breathe, you get rapid bursts of oxygen. This kicks in your *fight or flight system*. This is what it is there for. Unless there is a real reason to fight or flee, then shallow breathing is causing you undue stress and tension.

To reduce unnecessary stress and tension, and to return to our naturally calm state, we need to breathe deeply, from our belly. There is a specific point, in the Hara, known in Japanese, as the lower "Tan-Den". (The Tan-Den is called the Dan Tien in Chinese traditions) This point lies just below the navel. This remarkable point is where your vital spirit, has its centre. It is seems to correspond to your creative centre, otherwise known as the Sacral Chakra.

The ideal breath is to draw on the Ki of the Heavens, and the Earth. This is achieved by breathing with the Hara. Simply breathe deeply, into your lower abdomen, (three finger widths below your navel). Allow your belly to rise, as you inhale. Feel the energy of the breath, as it expands into your Hara. Draw your belly in, as you exhale, and allow the energy to circulate, throughout your entire body. At first, you may wish to place your palm on your Tan-Den, to get familiar with its rise and fall.

When you train your Hara, you strengthen your whole body, and bring calmness to your centre.

3) Meditating from your centre - We have already indicated that a calm mind, is also required so that the flow of Ki is not obstructed. This can be achieved through meditation. Typically, seated meditation is done in Lotus position where you have your legs crossed in front of you. The Lotus position is quite comfortable to some people, for others however, it may cause problems for their back, or legs. If, while in the Lotus position, you find it challenging to stop your hips from tilting backward, and that, in turn, causes your back to bend, then sitting on a Zazen pillow may help to provide a better angle between your back and your legs.

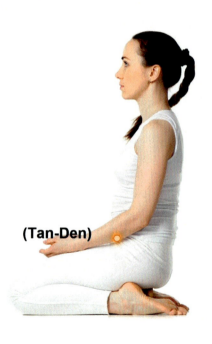
(Tan-Den)

I also recommend the Japanese meditation position called Seiza, as an alternative you may wish to try. This meditation position, allows you to sit with your legs under you. Your buttocks either sit on your heels or slip between your legs to the floor. You may also find it more comfortable, with a Zazen pillow between your legs, to sit on.

- Whichever way, you choose to sit, it is important to be comfortable, so you can meditate without strain on your back, and allow you to relax fully, in your chosen position.

- Your head should rest at an angle, with the infant soft spot of your skull (fontanelle), as the highest point. Your chin will be tilted slightly towards your chest.

- You may close your eyes, or sit with them slightly open. If slightly opened, gaze without interest, at a point on the floor, about five feet in front of you.

- Release your jaw so that it is relaxed and your teeth are slightly apart. Your lips will be closed as you touch the tip of your tongue to the roof of your mouth, just behind your teeth.

- Your hands should be at rest on your lap, or on your thighs.

- Begin to breathe into your Hara as taught above. Let your breath be your Guru. Focus completely on your breathing technique and on the CV 6 (Tan-Den) below your navel. As you focus on your centre allow your thoughts to come, and go as they please, without any attachment to them. Simply return to the breath as the space between your thoughts expands. Release all tension and assume Correct Posture.

- Practice this seated meditation until you feel calm and centred. When you are able to mediate from your centre easily in this seated position you, will be able to return to this *Zen state* in any position, and at any time you feel disturbed.

4) Consciously circulating Ki - The Microcosmic Orbit - In order to channel Ki throughout your body, with the intention of circulating it, you will learn next how to achieve the Microcosmic Orbit:

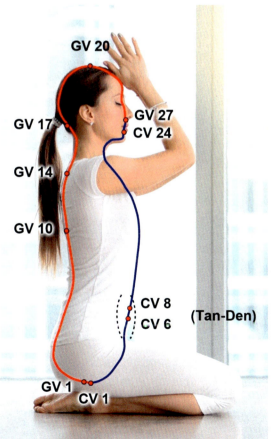

Once you have sufficiently practiced, Mediating from your Centre, and Breathing from your Hara, you will become quite aware, of the energetic build-up in your Hara. (It will feel quite warm and tingly.) Having achieved this, you are now ready to circulate the Ki, generated in your Hara, in what is called the Microcosmic orbit.

This orbit follows the path of two important meridian channels. The details of these meridians we will visit later, however, we will go over them briefly for this exercise.

Don't worry too much about memorizing the meridian points. It is the effect of the Microcosmic Orbit, that we are currently interested in experiencing.

The front vessel is called the **Conception Vessel** and contains the Yin energy circulation. For the purpose of the Microcosmic Orbit, this meridian starts at the lower lip, which point is called CV 24. It then passes down the front centreline, of the body, to a point at the perineum. (CV 1).

The back vessel is called the **Governing Vessel** and contains the Yang energy circulation. This meridian begins at your root point (GV 1), and travels up the centreline of your back, over the top of your head, down the centreline of your face, and ends at the roof of your mouth (GV 27).

These two vessels are not connected at this point. However, when the tongue, (called the Red Dragon), touches the roof of the mouth, it acts as a switch and completes the circuit. The tongue should not touch the teeth or the soft palette at the back but rest against the roof of the mouth. This bridge carries the flow of Ki from the Governing Vessel, to the Conception Vessel.

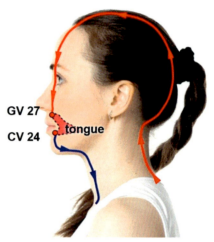

The circulation of Ki energy, in the Microcosmic Orbit, begins with the generation of energy in your Hara. This is achieved in the following way:

- Begin by sitting in Correct Posture, and relaxing completely.

- Breathe into your Hara, as taught, drawing the energy of the breath, deep into your belly, with each inhalation.

- Calm your mind, by Mediating from your Centre, making sure, that your tongue is set, against the roof of your mouth, (GV 27) just above and behind your teeth.

- The Tan-Den is known as the furnace. This is where you build up the fire. Feel this heat, building up in your belly, at the Tan-Den (CV 6). When the heat, and tingly sensations, are present in your belly, you can begin to consciously direct this energy.

- With your exhalation, direct the Ki down the Conception Vessel. It should travel from the CV 6, at the Hara, to the GV 1 point, at the perineum.

- The GV 1 point, at your Root, is where you squeeze to draw the energy up your back, on the next inhalation. **The trick to this is to tighten the anal sphincter while inhaling.**

- Continue to draw and inhale, the Ki flow up your back. Simply focus on the point, where you want the Ki to flow, and it will flow there, as long as you remain calm and relaxed.

- Guide the Ki, all the way up your back channel, and over the top of your head. As it passes over your head, you will feel a tingly sensation. Envision it flowing down over your face to GV 27.

- At this point, it passes through GV 28, on your upper lip, and reaches the Conception Vessel, at CV 24. Now exhale the Ki, down this front centreline channel, to your Hara, where the cycle starts over again.

Please Note: The flow is a continuous inhalation, from GV 1 to GV 28. The noted points along the path in the picture, are places that could interrupt Ki flow. The goal here is to clear the pathway, through these points, so you have an energetic Microcosmic Orbit, up the Governing Vessel, and down the Conception Vessel.

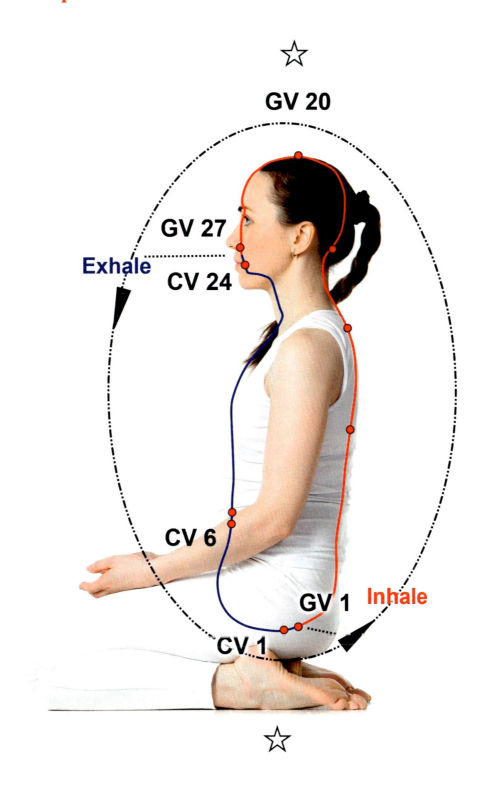

To summarize, the first four principles in Reikiatsu involved:

1. Letting go of tension in your body.
2. Deepening your breathing.
3. Calming your mind, though centre-focused meditation.
4. Circulating Ki, through the Microcosmic Orbit.

The above principles, were to prepare you to be, "in the zone", where you can consciously transport Ki. You have, undoubtedly, already had some experience with the feelings produced by directing Ki, while practicing Reiki. However, it is the intention of this book, that following these guidelines, will amplify the Ki flowing through you, and enhance your experience.

CIRCULATING THE FLOW OF KI THROUGH THE CHAKRAS:

For those of you, requiring a little assistance, in experiencing the Microcosmic Orbit, I would like to suggest the following exercise. After this exercise, we will move on to principle 5.

You are undoubtedly quite familiar, with the Chakra System, so we will approach the powerful circular flow of Ki energy, from this perspective.

There are 7 major chakras, beginning at your base with the Root Chakra. Once awakened, pranic energy passes upwards, from the Root Chakra, through a core channel, known as the Sushumna. This central energy channel, travels the full length of the spinal cord, and is the same channel, as the Governing vessel in the Microcosmic Orbit.

Approximately six inches, above your Crown Chakra, there is a little less known energy centre, called the Soul Star. Celestial/Spiritual/Cosmic energy, enters the body through this chakra.

Also. twelve or so inches, below your Root Chakra, is another energy centre, known as the Earth Star. This energy centre, grounds, or anchors you, to the magnetic core of mother earth.

With this understanding, we will begin our current exercise:

- Begin with sitting in your chosen Correct Posture, and relax completely.
- Breathe slowly and deeply into your Solar Plexus Chakra, drawing the energy of the breath into your belly, with each inhalation.
- Calm your mind, by mediating from your centre, making sure that your tongue is lightly touching, the roof of your mouth.
- Pay attention to your inhalations, and exhalations. Feel yourself expand, and deflate.
- Envision your Earth Star, about 12 inches, below your root.
- When you are ready, and your belly is warm, exhale, deflate, and direct the energy flow into the Earth Star. Pause, and feel the flow.

- Upon inhalation, expand and draw the energy, all the way up your back channel (Sushumna/Governing Vessel), to your Soul Star. Pause, and feel the flow.
- Upon the next exhalation, allow the energy to flow down, like a waterfall, over the front of your face, and body, all the way down, through your Root Chakra, to your Earth Star.
- Pause, then inhale the energy flow, up your back, once again, to your Soul Star.
- This, is the feeling you are after. When you establish this feeling, you can amplify the flow. Simply squeeze your root muscles as you inhale the Ki, up your back vessel, to the top of your head, through your Crown to your Soul Star.
- When you feel the sensations of the energetic flow, passing up, and down, your front and back centreline in a continuous loop, you have successfully initiated the Microcosmic Orbit!

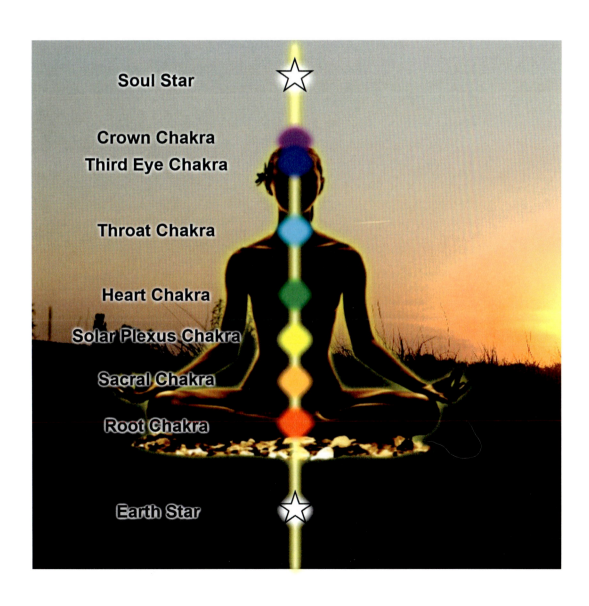

5) Consciously Directing Ki - The Macrocosmic Orbit

Before learning to transport Reiki, in a Reikiatsu Session, we are now going to practice, *Directing Ki into Infinity,* from the Macrocosmic Orbit. In this *Grand Circulation,* Ki passes through your entire body and returns to its Source. (All is One). When you tap into your connection with Source and are in harmony with it, the yin and yang of appearances, are in balance.

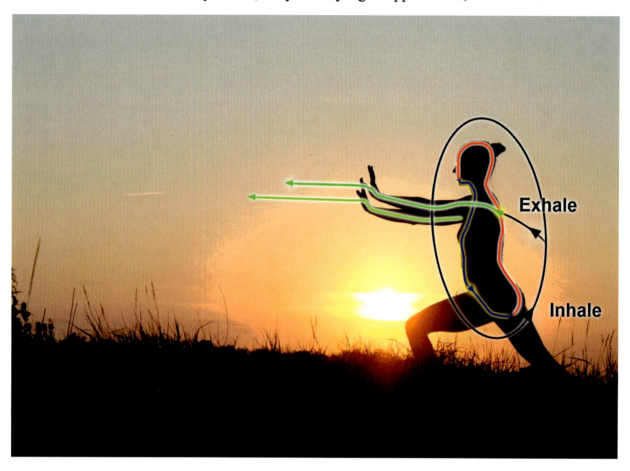

Directing Ki into Infinity is simply circulating the flow of Ki, throughout your entire meridian system, and then, consciously transporting it, to the Infinite Source of All. The grand circulation of Ki, through all your meridians, is called the Macrocosmic Orbit. Directing Ki to Infinity, will be learned, as you follow these guidelines:

- Begin as you did, in the Microcosmic Orbit. Breath deep, and rhythmically, with the Ki following the path, up the Governing Vessel, through your back, and down the Conception Vessel, over the front of your body.

- Feel the tingling sensations, moving over, and though, your body, as the Ki circulates.

- Continue the microcosmic loop, but, as you do, begin to consciously direct, some of the flow, into your arms. Allow yourself to experience the sensations.

- Feel the flow of Ki build up in your hands. You can play with this energy. You can form it into a ball of energy that can be experienced between your hands.
- Now, experiment with directing the flow of Ki, into your legs, feet, and toes.
- Send this flow to different areas in your body. Take your time with this. Enjoy this journey of energetic, Self-discovery.
- When you feel confident that you can consciously intend and direct Ki, to your arms, legs, or other areas, you are successfully channelling Ki in the Macrocosmic Orbit.
- Having achieved this, you are ready to direct and transport Ki, to infinity.
- During an inhalation, draw the Ki up your back, as you have learned. At the point where it reaches shoulder level, envision the energy flowing forward, out, and through, your arms.
- Begin your exhale. Ki will still circulate, over the top of your head, but the powerful flow of Rei-ki energy will pass through your arms, and hands, as well.
- As you exhale, envision the Ki energy, being consciously "pushed", though your arms, and reaching to infinity. You will feel a great surge passing through you, as this happens.
- ***(Note: This pushing intention is the pressure, or as in Japanese, "atsu", whether you are, actually, physically, in contact or not.)***
- If you get side-tracked, simply return to a state of calmness, deepen your breathing, and draw the energy, up your channel again.

When you inhale you receive, and when you exhale you give.

This is the yin, and yang, of the rhythm of life.

NOTE: The idea of directing the Ki to infinity may seem a bit presumptuous, however, you are already familiar with Long Distance Reiki, and this is the same principle.

In Long Distance Reiki, you have a set location in your mind that you are sending the energy to. In consciously directing Ki to infinity, you are able to transcend all time and space.

To facilitate this, you can simply pick a point, let's say, 20 feet, and begin sending it there. You could also pick a location, another city, or a particular person, and send it there. Then, simply direct the energy, with your exhalation, beyond this point. Imagine it travelling, through and beyond the particular point, to a place, where there are no limitations.

An easy way to practice this is to send the energy the 20 feet, and then double it, to 40. Double it over, and over, until you see, that there is no end, to doubling it. Then, you suddenly realize, that even though, the Ki flow is being sent to infinity, it still, passes through the point, at 20 feet, 40 feet, 80 feet, and so on. Infinity is connected, to all places, and all points.

CHAPTER 2

THE MERIDIAN SYSTEM

The function of the human body Meridian System is to circulate Ki throughout the body. When the free flow of Ki is interrupted, this can lead to a lack of energy (Kyo) in one area and a surplus of energy (Jitsu) in another.

These blockages may be caused by stress, injury, traumatic experience, or unhealthy habits. Removing these blockages, through Ki flow stimulation or sedation, can balance the human body meridian system, and restore physical, mental and spiritual health.

"Supply energy where there is deficiency and sedate energy when there is an excess."
~ The Yellow Emperor's Classic of Internal Medicine

THE 14 MAIN HUMAN BODY MERIDIANS

For the purpose of directing Ki into and through the meridians and their points, we have to acquire a basic knowledge of the fourteen main meridians. *Do not try to memorize all the points, etc., or you may find it overwhelming at this stage. We will cover the impact of each meridian, more specifically, in the section devoted to Reikatsu Sessions.*

For now, we need to know that there are Fourteen Main Meridians that flow throughout the human body. Twelve of these are paired and complement each other with Yin energy flowing upwards, and Yang energy flowing downwards. The remaining Two Meridians are single, centrally located, channels that flow into each other.

The twelve primary pairs that consist of six yang and six yin meridians are:

- The Stomach Meridian (Yang) is paired with the Spleen Meridian (Yin).
- The Heart Meridian (Yin) is paired with the Small Intestine Meridian (Yang).
- The Bladder Meridian (Yang) is paired with the Kidney Meridian (Yin).
- The Pericardium Meridian (Yin), is paired with Triple Heater Meridian (Yang).
- The Gallbladder Meridian (Yang) is paired with the Liver Meridian (Yin).
- The Lung Meridian (Yin), is paired with the Large Intestine Meridian (Yang).

The two single centrally located meridians are:

- The Governing Vessel (Yang) which flows into the Conception Vessel (Yin).

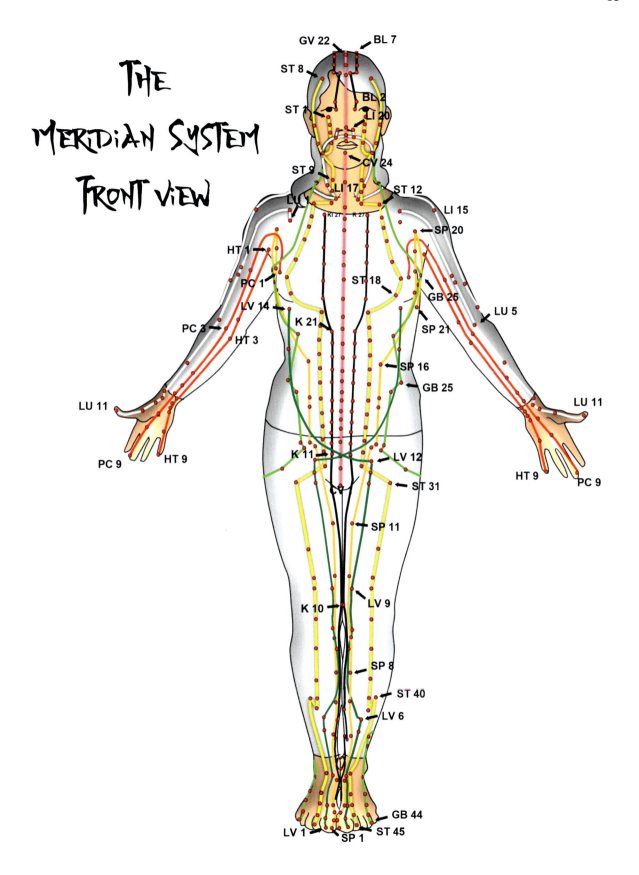

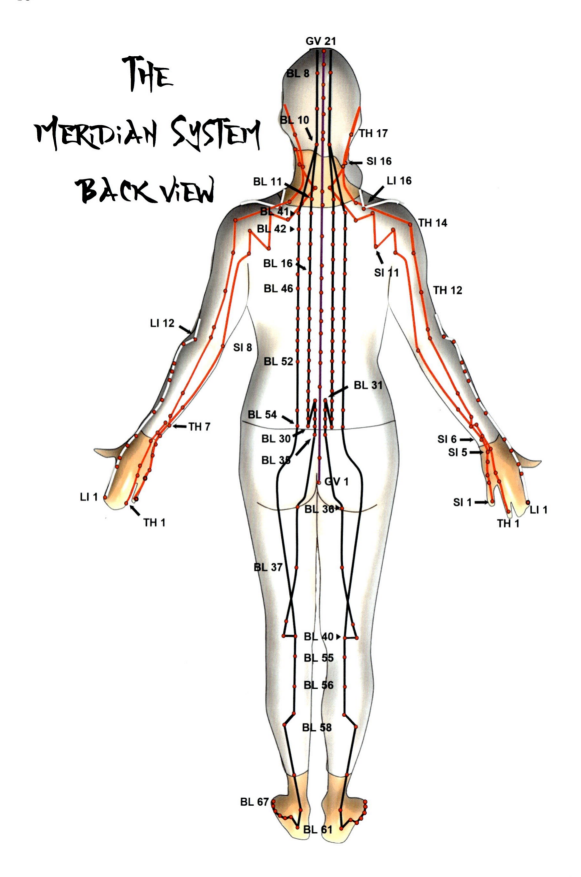

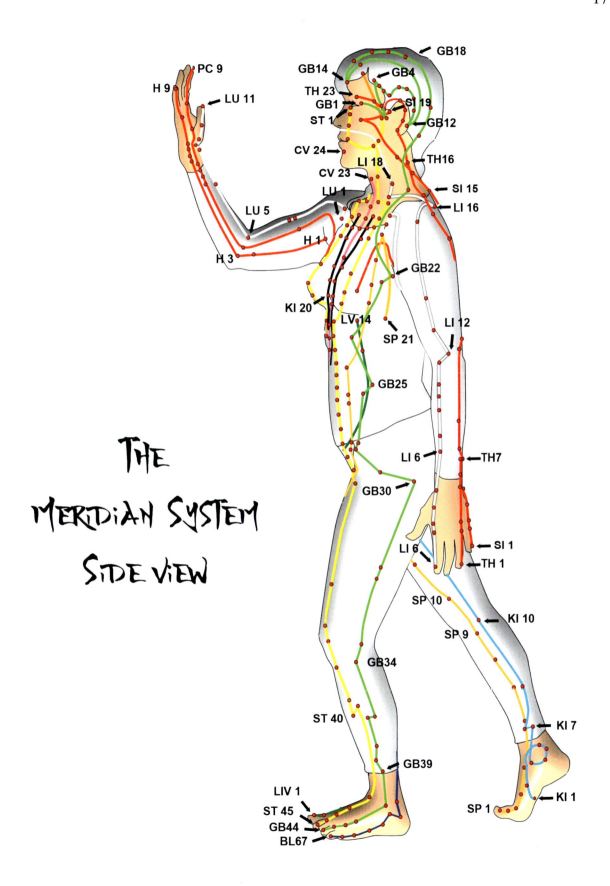

THE STOMACH MERIDIAN

Known as the *Sea of Nourishment,* the Stomach Meridian's primary function is to provide physical and emotional nourishment. When the body and emotions are adequately nourished, we are dynamic, compassionate, and confident beings with the capacity to nurture others. When the stomach meridian Ki is balanced, we are able to experience empathy through our deep connection to the core of mother earth.

Physically, the stomach is responsible for the digestion and absorption of food. Energetically, it functions with the spleen in transporting the Ki obtained from food, through the meridian system to the lungs, where it combines with the Ki obtained from oxygen.

The Stomach Meridian (Yang) is paired with the Spleen Meridian (Yin).

Ki Flow Direction: ↓ Down

- **Stomach Meridian Element:** The stomach is governed by the Earth, an element with strong nurturing qualities. It is responsible for extracting and balancing all five elemental energies obtained from foods and fluids. Any imbalance of the stomach energy ends up in an imbalance in the Ki channelled from the stomach to other organs.
- **Physical Imbalances:** These imbalances in energy show up, physically, as digestive and stomach disorders such as abdominal cramps, bloating, vomiting, and even sore throats.
- **Emotional Imbalances:** When the Ki of the stomach meridian is imbalanced it may appear as anxiety attacks, insecurity, feelings of abandonment, distrust, and self-centeredness.
- **Peak Hours:** 7 a.m. - 9 a.m.
- **Ascribed Colour:** Yellow
- **Location:** Beginning at ST 1, between the lower eyelid and the eye socket, the stomach meridian travels down the face and then swings up to the side of the forehead. At ST 8, it then travels back down the channel. This time, it travels down the neck and across to the indent just above the midpoint of the collar bone. It then travels down the ribs, to just below the nipple. It then moves to a point lateral to the centreline of the body and travels down the ribs and over the abdomen. When it reaches a point at the height of the pubic area, it moves across to ST 31 at the top of the leg. It travels down the leg ending at ST 45, on the outside edge of the second toe.

Transformational Affirmation:

I trust in the Light of the Universe to support and nourish my every need.

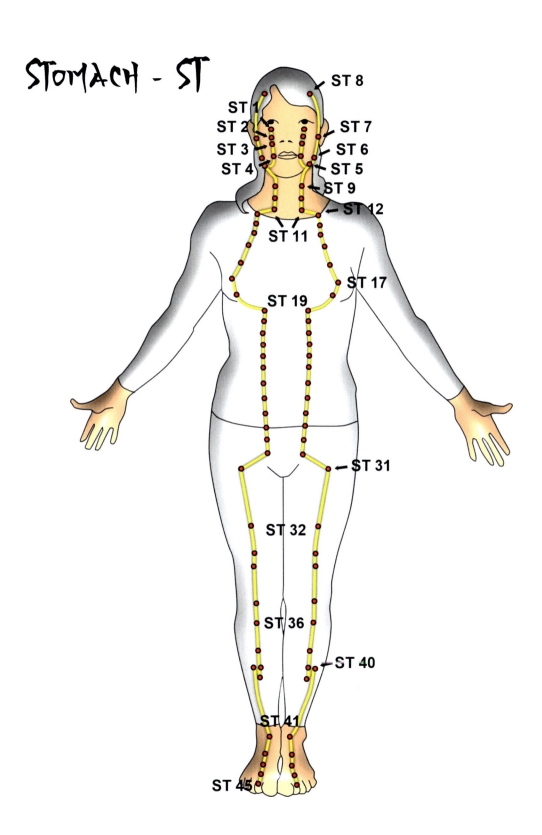

THE SPLEEN MERIDIAN

Known as the *Minister of the Granary*, the Spleen Meridian is involved in the restoration of self-esteem and empowerment.

The spleen organ energy system includes the pancreas. The spleen is responsible for the removal of old red blood cells and the production and storage of white blood cells (lymphocytes) which will cleanse bacteria from the blood in the spleen and provide tissue restoration, and other immune responses throughout our body.

The spleen is the principal organ involved in the transformation of water and food into the Ki and blood of the body.

The Spleen Meridian (Yin) is paired with the Stomach Meridian (Yang).

Ki Flow Direction: ↑ Up

- **Spleen Meridian Element:** The spleen is also governed by the Earth, an element with strong nurturing qualities. If the body is well nourished, our muscles and limbs will be strong.

- **Physical Imbalances:** These disturbances show up as digestive and stomach problems, weak limbs and muscle atrophy.

- **Emotional Imbalances:** Indications of blockages or imbalances show up as worry, hopelessness, poor concentration, forgetfulness, addictions, living vicariously through others, jealousy, self-pity, low self-esteem, etc..

- **Peak Hours:** 9 a.m. - 11 a.m.

- **Ascribed Colour:** Yellow

- **Location:** The spleen meridian begins on the inside of the foot at the tip of the big toe. From there it runs along the inner aspect of the foot. It then travels up the inner leg, just behind the leg bone, up to the groin. From there it runs up the abdomen, through the diaphragm, and over the chest. At SP 20, a point in the space under the second rib, it travels down to the outside of the chest to a point in the space under the 6th rib (SP 21). (At SP 20 this meridian also branches out, internally, to reach the throat and root of the tongue, although there are no points along this path.)

Transformational Affirmation:

I embrace a sense of compassion for myself, as I process and use all that I experience.

SPLEEN - SP

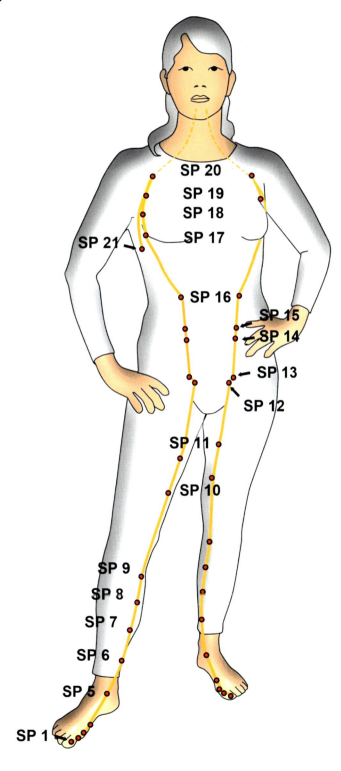

THE HEART MERIDIAN

The Heart Meridian is recognized as the *King of the Organs*. It is said, *"The heart commands all of the organs and viscera, houses the spirit, and controls the emotions"*.

The heart rules the circulation and distribution of blood. Therefore, all of the body depends upon it for sustenance. It has dominion over the blood, tongue, throat, sweat, facial complexion, adrenals, thyroid, prostate and pituitary gland.

To live from the heart is to recognize the heart's innate intelligence. This is the Governor that rules in the House of the Spirit. It is the Mind of our Heart that reveals itself through the light in our eyes.

The Heart Meridian (Yin) is paired with the Small Intestine Meridian (Yang).

Ki Flow Direction: ↑ Up

- **Heart Meridian Element:** The Heart Meridian belongs to the Fire element. Fire is associated with warmth, laughter, and enthusiasm. This blaze of Fire is summer's energetic gift, that allows us to give and receive warmth. Through giving and sharing, we build our own Fire, open our own flower, and bring more of the summer sun to the world. Nowhere is the warmth of love felt more deeply than in the Heart.

- **Physical Imbalances:** Experiences of a shortness of breath, coldness in the chest and limbs, palpitations, cold sweat, the inability to speak, memory failure and restless sleep.

- **Emotional Imbalances:** The heart is the ruler of all emotions. Signs of imbalance include agitation, sadness, the excess or an absence of laughter, depression, fear, anxiety, inconsistent behaviour, loneliness, jealousy, and sorrow.

- **Peak Hours:** 11 a.m. - 1 p.m.

- **Ascribed Colour:** Red

- **Location:** This meridian starts at the heart and divides into three branches. One passes down internally, through the diaphragm to the small intestine. Another internal branch moves up through the throat to the eye, with a connection to the tongue. A third branch goes internally to the lung before it surfaces at the centre of the armpit. From here the heart meridian descends along the inner side of the arm. It continues down to the inner tip of the little finger. (This meridian only has points, once it surfaces, from H 1 to H 9).

Transformational Affirmation:

My heart awakens and is open to receive and transmit unconditional love.

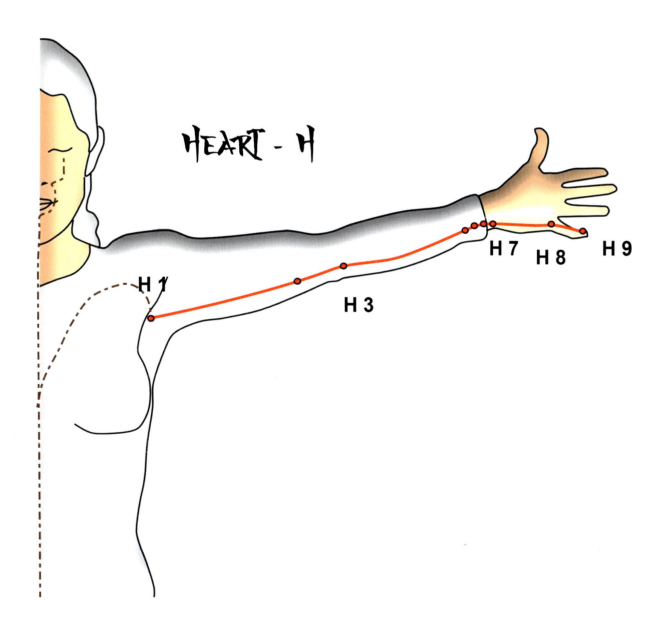

THE SMALL INTESTINE MERIDIAN

Known as the *Minister of Reception*, this meridian receives and distinguishes between the pure and the impure. It is involved in determining what is essential and good for you.

The small intestine is a semi-permeable barrier that receives partially digested food from the stomach and refines it even more, separating the desirable nutrients from the undesirable waste. It then assimilates the purified nutrients and moves the impure wastes onwards to the urinary bladder, kidneys and large intestine for elimination. This meridian is responsible for digestion, water absorption, nutrient absorption and bowel functions.

The Small Intestine Meridian (Yang) is paired with the Heart Meridian (Yin).

Ki Flow Direction: ↓ Down

- **Small Intestine Element:** Associated with the heart, the small intestine meridian also belongs to Fire energy. Energetically, the small intestine impacts the more basic emotions. Its meridian also runs into the head, where it affects the function of the pituitary gland, whose secretions regulate growth, metabolism, immunity, sexuality, and the entire endocrine system.

- **Physical Imbalances:** Signs include digestive and elimination problems such as abdominal pain, constipation, diarrhea, too much, or too little urination, as well as hearing issues, including tinnitus.

- **Emotional Imbalances:** These are indicated by a lack of mental clarity that manifests as an inability to evaluate or assimilate ideas. It also shows up as a fear of commitment, vulnerability, cynical thinking, insecurity, or sarcasm.

- **Peak Hours:** 1 p.m. - 3 p.m.

- **Ascribed Colour:** Red

- **Location:** The Small Intestine Meridian starts at the outside tip of the little fingernail and runs up the outside of the hand to the wrist. It then runs upwards along the posterior side of the forearm until it reaches the back of shoulder where it ends at the uppermost part of the back, at the bottom of the neck. (An internal branch travels down from here over the shoulder through the heart and stomach to the small intestine). At this position, it also travels externally across the neck to the cheek then ends in front of the ear.

Transformational Affirmation:

I trust my ability to know what is good for me, and I make healthy decisions for myself.

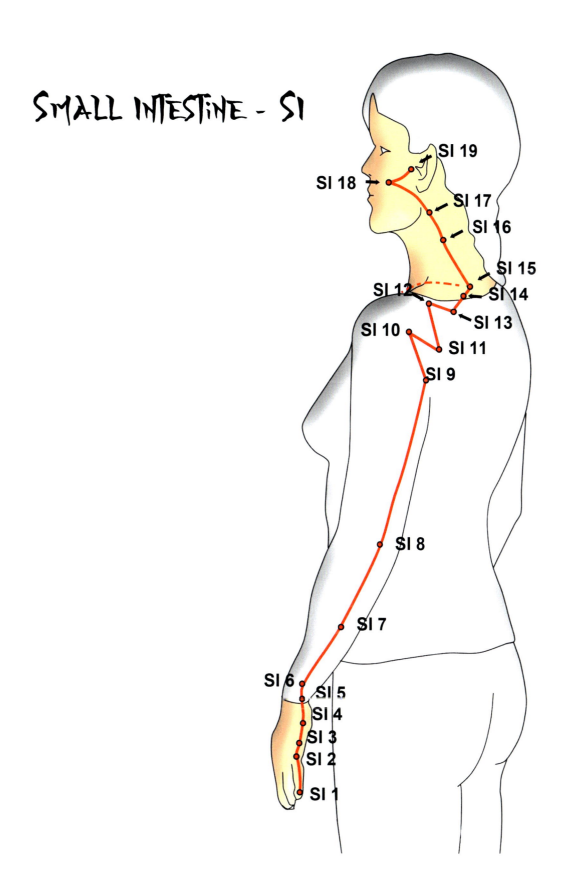

THE BLADDER MERIDIAN

The Bladder Meridian is known as the *Minister of the Reservoir,* and energetically, it is the reservoir for your daily supply of Ki. It counsels you to slow down and to rest so that you don't deplete your energy reserves.

The urinary bladder is responsible for storing and excreting the urinary waste fluids passed down from the kidneys. This meridian governs the autonomic nervous system.

The Bladder Meridian (Yang) is paired with the Kidney Meridian (Yin).

Ki Flow Direction: ↓ Down

- **Bladder Meridian Element:** Associated with the kidney, the bladder meridian belongs to Water Energy a powerful and creative force centred in the lower abdomen. The Water Element is the element of winter and manifests as the power of will, ambition, determination, perseverance, and resolve. These qualities arise from having a full reservoir of Ki.

- **Physical Imbalances:** These include headaches, back problems (especially around the kidneys), urinary problems including excessive urination and incontinence, as well as other issues involving fluid movement in the body.

- **Emotional Imbalances:** These manifest as a lack of energy, feeling overwhelmed, smothered, empty, or fearful. A lack of hope is common.

- **Peak Hours:** 3 p.m. - 5 p.m.

- **Ascribed Colour:** Blue/Black

- **Location:** This long, complex meridian begins at the inside corner of the eyelid and travels up to the eyebrow, across the forehead, to the hairline. It then moves across laterally and passes over the scalp to the back of the head. At BL 10 it forms two branches that travel down the back beside the spine, all the way to the sacrum. Please Note: This meridian travels down along side the spine from BL 11 to BL 30, moves up beside the sacrum to BL 31, and then travels down the sacrum to BL 35, over the buttocks to BL 36, and moves on down the legs to BL 40. The second branch travels down on the outer channel beside the spine and is numbered from BL 41 to the knee point BL 54. It then also passes over the buttocks, where two branches pass over the back of thigh along their separate paths until they join behind the knee. The now single meridian travels down from BL 55 and over the calves to the Achilles tendon where it moves to the outside of the foot. The bladder meridian ends here, on the outside of the little toe.

Transformational Affirmation:

I believe in my potential to achieve my goals. The future looks bright.

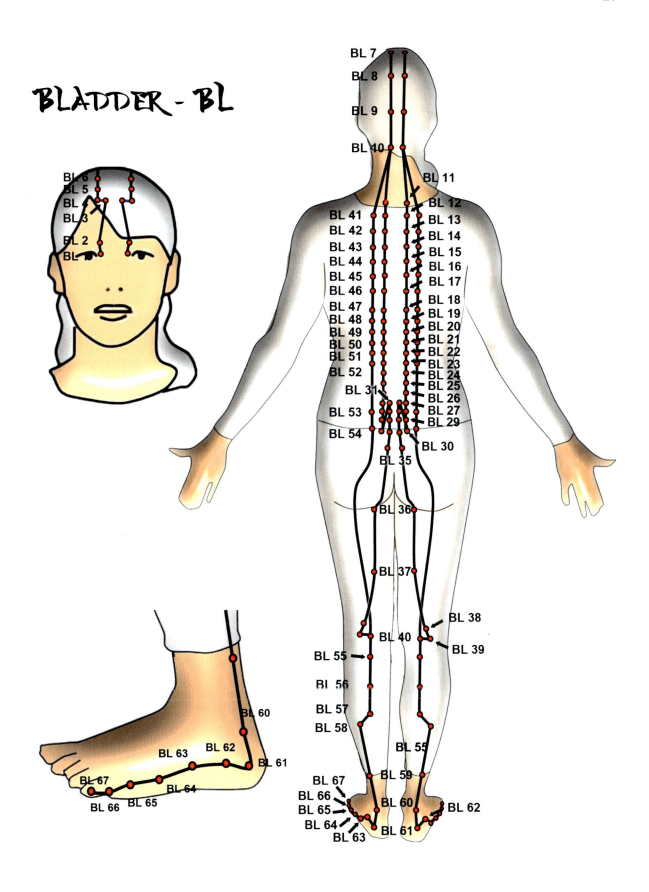

THE KIDNEY MERIDIAN

Known as the *Minister of Power,* the Kidney Meridian is regarded as *Seat of Courage and Willpower*. This Meridian is considered the source of the body's constitutional energy that governs the integrity and function not only of the kidneys themselves, but also rules over the ovaries, testes, adrenal glands, brain, spinal cord, skeletal structure, teeth, anus, urethra, and inner ear as well. The Kidney system also governs body fluids, vital tissues, hormones and other substances produced by the kidneys. Adrenals and sex glands, reproduction, growth and the faculty of will power, are impacted by this meridian as well..

The kidneys are responsible for filtering metabolic wastes from the blood and directing them to the bladder for excretion in urine. Working with the large intestine, the kidneys control the balance of fluids in the body. They also regulate the body's acid-alkaline balance by filtering out or retaining a variety of minerals.

The Kidney Meridian (Yin) is paired with the Bladder Meridian (Yang).

Ki Flow Direction: ↑ Up

- **Kidney Meridian Element:** As with the bladder meridian, the Kidney Meridian is associated with the Water Element. This is the element that corresponds to winter, and directs us to that dark, quiet pool within ourselves where our true essence resides. It is a time for deep, inner work. Meditation, quiet contemplation and the restoring of our energy are the objectives of the water element..

- **Physical Imbalances:** One affected by an imbalance in this meridian may experience anemia, chest pain, asthma, abdominal pain, irregular menstruation, or impotence.

- **Emotional Imbalances:** These may show up as hysteria, paranoia, depression, fear, loneliness and insecurity. Anxiety, or panic attacks may be experienced.

- **Peak Hours:** 5 p.m. - 7 p.m.

- **Ascribed Colour:** Blue/Black

- **Location:** This meridian begins under the little toe, and passes through KI 1 to the inside edge of the foot. Looping behind the inside if the ankle bone towards the heel, it then travels along the inside of the the calf and thigh. At the top of the inner thigh it runs deeper towards the sacrum, where it joins the governing vessel. (Rising internally, it enters the kidney, then travels to the surface at the pubic area.) It then ascends externally over the front of the body to the collarbone.

Transformational Affirmation:

I am gentle with myself as I step out of my comfort zone and accomplish what is required of me.

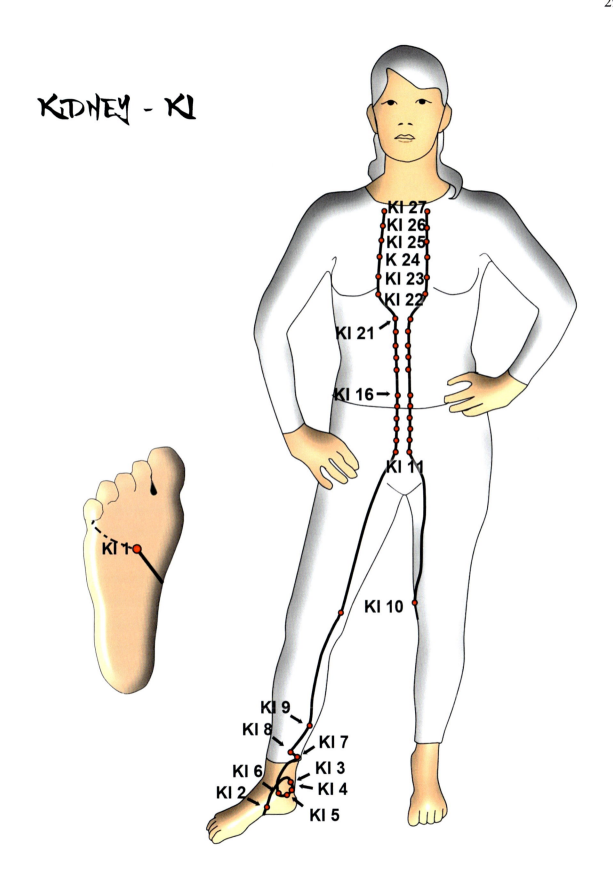

THE PERICARDIUM MERIDIAN

Known as the *King's Bodyguard,* the Pericardium Meridian is regarded as the heart's protector.

When the heart is not well protected, our ability to express love and experience joy is compromised. We forget our connection to Spirit and feel all alone. When the King's Bodyguard is balanced and strong, it protects us from harm and opens to healthy, positive, and rewarding relationships.

The pericardium is a double-walled sac enveloping and protecting the heart, as well as the roots of the major blood vessels. It consists of an outer fibrous layer and an inner double layer of serous membrane.

The Pericardium Meridian (Yin) is also called the Heart Constrictor or Circulation-Sex Meridian. It is paired with the Triple Heater Meridian (Yang) that is also sometimes known as the Triple Energizer or Triple Burner Meridian.

Ki Flow Direction: ↑ Up

- **Pericardium Meridian Element:** The Pericardium Meridian is associated with the Fire Element. As with the Heart, Small Intestine and Triple Heater meridians, this Fire Element meridian is associated with the summer. Summertime displays its natural power in full bloom. Only at summertime's peak do plants spread pollen to propagate more of their kind. Only mature animals reproduce. It is Summer's act of expressing love that is an expressions of the Fire element. It is the deep love within summer's Fire, that we fully open to the passion, warmth, and joy, of truly intimate relationships.

- **Physical Imbalances**: When the Ki of the Pericardium Meridian is out of balance, a person may experience various disorders of the chest area, including chest pain, heart palpitations, angina, or anxiety attacks.

- **Emotional Imbalances:** An imbalanced Pericardium Meridian will show up emotionally as feeling lonely, exhausted, abandoned, depressed, unappreciated or invisible.

- **Peak Hours: 7** p.m. - 9 p.m.

- **Ascribed Colour:** Red

- **Location:** The Pericardium Meridian begins in the middle of the chest. An internal branch travels down through the diaphragm. It also branches out from the centre of the chest at the pericardium, and crosses the chest to surface just outside the nipples. It then runs around the front of the armpit and flows down the inner surface of the arm. It ends at the tip of the middle finger.

Transformational Affirmation:

My acute sense of discernment allows me to guard against all that is not in harmony with my highest good. I exercise my ability to choose for myself those experiences that fill me with the fire of love and passion.

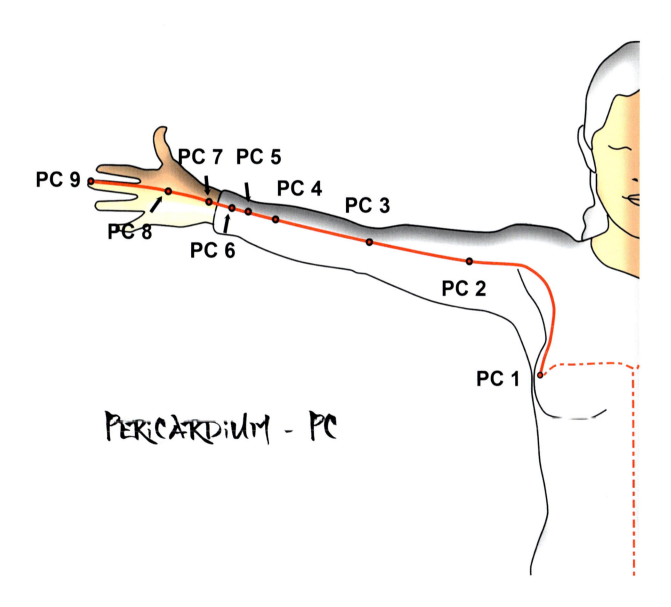

PERICARDIUM - PC

THE TRIPLE HEATER MERIDIAN

This Meridian is also known as the Triple Burner, Triple Warmer, or Triple Energizer Meridian. Considered to be the *Minister of Dykes and Dredges* or the *Officer of Balance and Harmony*, the Triple Heater Meridian is in charge of the transformation and flow of Ki in the body.

The Triple Heater balances the body's energy by regulating its temperature, and by metabolizing our bodily fluids. Having been separated by the spleen into pure and waste fluids, the Triple Heater's upper, middle and lower burners are responsible for the intake, transformation, and elimination of these fluids. Although there is no physical organ associated with this meridian, these three burners are located as:

- The Upper - heart/lungs known as *The Mist*.
- The Middle - stomach/spleen/liver/gall bladder/small intestine, known as *The Foam*.
- The Lower - kidney/bladder/large intestine, known as *The Swamp*.

The Triple Heater Meridian (Yang) is paired with the Pericardium Meridian (Yin).

Ki Flow Direction: ↓ Down

- **Triple Heater Meridian Element:** The element of Fire is associated with the peak of summer. This is a time when opportunities abound for many activities. Being highly active during this time is conducive to cleansing our system. The warmth of summer's activities activates sweating and the release of toxins. The burning off of these fluids allows the Ki to flow unobstructed. The outcome of this is a clearing of the mind of toxic residues such as prejudices and discrimination.

- **Physical Imbalances:** Imbalances in the Ki flowing through this meridian result in headaches, especially in the temples, as well as ear issues. An imbalance in the Ki of this meridian can also show up as feeling flushed, fevers, chills, hot flashes and night sweats.

- **Emotional Imbalances:** An imbalance here results in the inability to "burn off" toxic thoughts. One may experience fear inducing chronic fight/flight/freeze impulses. Suspiciousness in all relationships is a sign of Ki imbalances in this meridian.

- **Peak Hours:** 9 p.m. - 11 p.m.

- **Ascribed Colour:** Red

- **Location:** The Triple Heater Meridian begins at the tip of the ring finger and travels up the hand between the knuckles of the fourth and fifth fingers. At the wrist, it runs between the two bones of the forearm, and upward through the tip of the elbow. It then moves up the back of the arm to the shoulder. At the upper angle of the scapula, the meridian ascends up the side of the neck and around to the back of the ear.

Transformational Affirmation:

I trust in the Light of the Universe to keep me safe and secure.

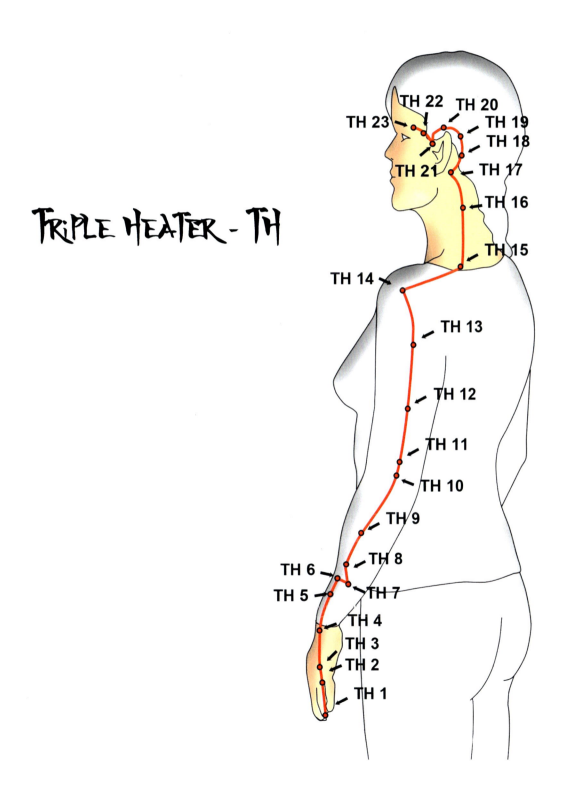

THE GALLBLADDER MERIDIAN

Known as the *Honourable Minister*, the Gallbladder Meridian is responsible for the Ki that is utilized in our decision making processes, and the ability to make good choices. It provides the courage and initiative to follow through with our decisions.

Physically, the gallbladder secretes the digestive enzyme, bile, that is required to digest and metabolize fats and oils. It also breaks up fats and works with the lymphatic system to clear toxins from the muscular system. It thereby, assists in eliminating muscular aches and fatigue.

The Gallbladder Meridian (Yang) is paired with the Liver Meridian (Yin).

Ki Flow Direction: ↓ Down

- **Gallbladder Meridian Element:** Wood is associated with the Gallbladder Meridian. The Wood element contributes to the clarity of mind when envisioning goals, and making them come to life. This process is all about being clear of obstacles and toxicity that would impair forward and free movement.

- **Physical Imbalances:** When the Ki flow is weak, and this channel is out of balance, sleeping patterns are affected. Elimination issues may be a result and show up as bloating, constipation or diarrhea, etc..

- **Emotional Imbalances:** Persons with an imbalance here may be given to various addictions. These poor choices may be compulsive tendencies that appear as ways to deal with feelings of resentment, a lack of passion, repression, depression, and indecisiveness. Fits of anger and blame usually accompany these emotions.

- **Peak Hours:** 11 p.m. - 1 a.m.

- **Ascribed Colour:** Green

- **Location:** The Gallbladder Meridian originates just outside the outer corner of the eye and travels downwards towards to the depression in front of the ear. It then runs up the forehead to the hairline. It travels down behind the ear to the corner of the skull, before returning to the forehead, above the centre of the eye. From there it over the top of the head along the side of the centreline, and travels down to the base of the skull. Travelling down the neck to the shoulder, it then descends to just in front of the armpit. From there it runs down the side of the body over the ribs, to the waist and pelvis. From GB 30, between the tailbone and the top of the leg bone, it runs down the outside of the leg, to the ankle, and ends on the outside edge of the 4th toe.

Transformational Affirmation:

I extend kindness and forgiveness in all my encounters. I am inspired to follow my bliss.

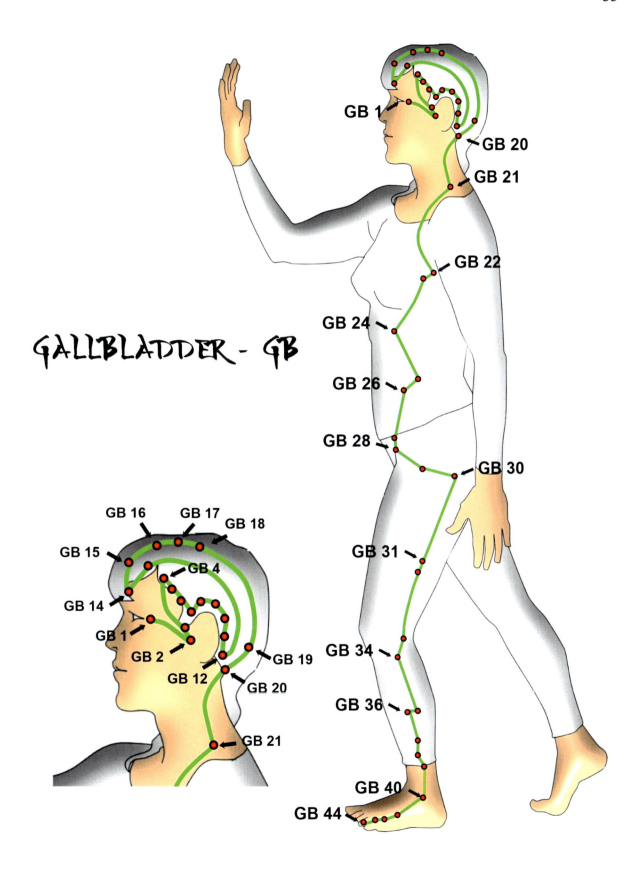

THE LIVER MERIDIAN

The liver is known as the *General*, or *Chief of Staff*, and oversees the replenishment of blood for growth and regeneration. This includes our growth and development as a person, since the liver meridian Ki is directly involved with the level of our drive, ambitions, and creativity.

As an organ, the liver governs the filtration, detoxification, nourishment, replenishment and storage of blood. The liver stores glycogen, a form of sugar, that is released into the blood as glucose whenever the body needs extra energy. The liver also receives all amino acids extracted from food. It then synthesizes these amino acids into various forms of protein required for the growth and renewal of body tissues.

The Liver Meridian (Yin) is paired with the Gallbladder Meridian (Yang).

Ki Flow Direction: ↑ Up

- **Liver Meridian Element**: Wood is the element associated with the Liver Meridian. This element empowers people that are balanced, to have clear ideas and visions about what they want to accomplish. They also have clarity about how to bring their desires into form. Their opinions are strong and they don't give in easily.

- **Physical Imbalances**: Liver Meridian imbalance, or weakness, manifests physically as eye problems and could show up as blurry vision. Brittle fingernails are also a sign of Liver Meridian imbalances.

- **Emotional Imbalances**: A person with an imbalance in the Liver Meridian will have less drive and tend to be weak in ambition. Blockages in energy here can cause irrational anger, and resentment, especially towards one's self. Self-sabotage is a common experience.

- **Peak Hours:** 1 a.m. - 3 a.m.

- **Ascribed Colour**: Green

- **Location:** The liver meridian originates at the inside edge of the big toe. It then travels over the top of the foot, in front of the inside ankle bone. Moving up the inside of the leg bone, it continues past the knee, and along the inside of the thigh to the groin. At this point, it curves over the genitals, across the pubic area, and up the lower abdomen to end just below the breast.

Transformational Affirmation:

I accept and appreciate all that I am. I release self-judgement and anger.

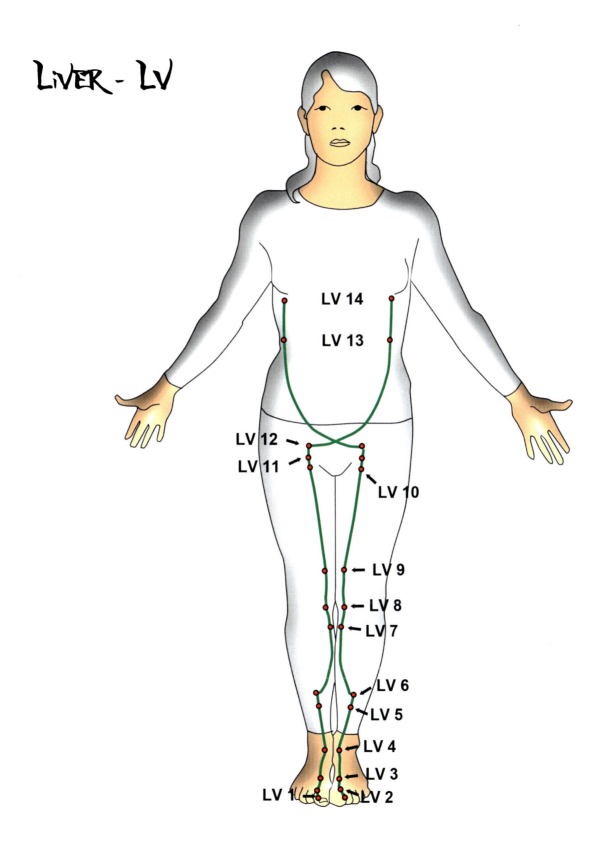

THE LUNG MERIDIAN

Known as, *the High Priest of Heaven,* the Lung Meridian is responsible for establishing the foundation of Ki for the entire body. In an intimate relationship with the heart, the lungs regulate the breath, and pulse. Energetically, the lungs oversee self-protection and self-preservation.

Breathing controls cellular respiration. Shallow and irregular breathing patterns contribute to lowered vitality and insufficient metabolism. The lungs also are involved with the skin, which by breathing through its pores, through perspiration, and shivering, assists in regulating the body's temperature. Breathing also directly impacts the autonomic nervous system. For this reason, breathing techniques are traditionally included as an integral part of yoga, tai chi, chi kung, and various forms of meditation. By consciously regulating the breath, the autonomic nervous system, the body's energy, and pulse, are brought into balance and harmony with the mind.

The Lung Meridian (Yin) is paired with the Large Intestine Meridian (Yang).

Ki Flow Direction: ↑ Up

- **Lung Meridian Element:** As the High Priest, the Lung Meridian receives and embraces the pure Ki of the heavens. This meridian is associated with the element of metal. This element speaks to us of the letting go of that which is old and stale, and opening up to the crisp, clear air of autumn. A person whose lung meridian Ki is flowing freely, releases what no longer serves without experiencing excessive grief. Just as precious metal elements have become a symbol of material wealth, so too, our sense of self-worth is based on the flow of the metal element Ki within our system. A person with a balanced lung meridian feels the abundance of mother earth flowing through them.

- **Physical Imbalances:** An imbalance of Ki flowing through the lung meridian shows up as various conditions in the chest, lung, throat and nose. Asthma, sinusitis, allergies, and the common cold are symptomatic. The lung meridian metal element also governs the skin, so an imbalance can appear in the form of rashes, eczema, and other skin related issues. As the lung meridian is paired with the meridian of the large intestine an imbalance may show up as chronic constipation, diarrhea, or other bowel-related illnesses.

- **Emotional Imbalances:** A blockage or imbalance in the lung meridian results in a person experiencing severe disappointment, grief, despair, anxiety, shame, and jealousy. They will feel betrayed and hang desperately onto the past, or material items, for a sense of worth.

- **Peak Hours:** 3 a.m. - 5 a.m.

- **Ascribed Colour:** White/silver

- **Location:** This meridian begins (internally) deep in the solar plexus region and descends to meet the large intestine meridian. Winding up past the stomach, it crosses the diaphragm, divides, and enters the lungs. It then reunites, passes up the middle of the windpipe to the throat and divides again, surfacing in the hollow region near the front of the shoulder (LU 1). From here it (externally) passes over the shoulder and down the front of the arm, along the outside of the biceps muscle. It then travels down the forearm to the wrist, just above the base of the thumb, and ends at the corner of the thumbnail.

Transformational Affirmation:

I release all that is not in harmony with my health and happiness. I let go of all that would cause me sorrow.

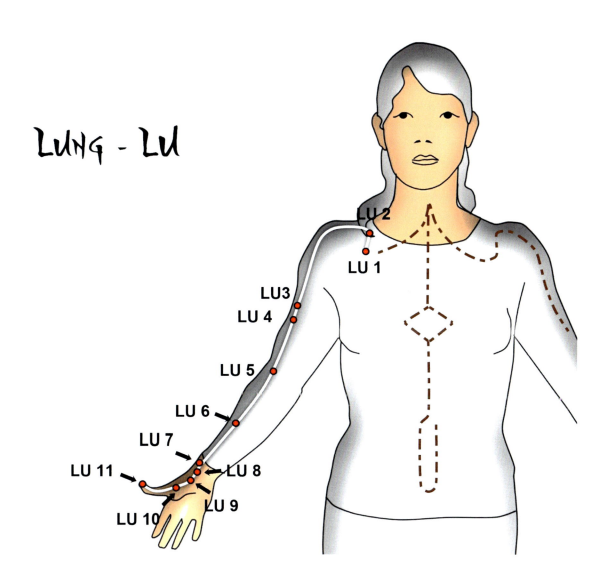

THE LARGE INTESTINE MERIDIAN

Called the *Minister of Transportation,* the Large Intestine Meridian governs our ability to discern and let go of what needs to move on and out of our lives. Discretion is required if we are to release ideas, and beliefs, that have us sluggish and bogged down.

Physically, the large intestine reabsorbs water from indigestible food and transports the useless waste material out of our body. It also plays a significant role in maintaining the balance and purity of our bodily fluids. It is also involved with the lungs in governing the skin's elimination of fluids through perspiration.

The Large Intestine Meridian (Yang) is paired with the Lung Meridian (Yin).

Ki Flow Direction: ↓ Down

- **Large Intestine Meridian Element:** Metal is the element of release, and calls us to let go of all that is not in harmony with our well being.

- **Physical Imbalances:** Paired with the lungs, the large intestine depends on the lungs for movement through the expansion and contraction of the diaphragm. This works like a pump creating waves of muscle contractions that moves along food to be processed. Sluggish bowels may be stimulated by belly breathing and by strengthening lung energy. Lung congestion or bronchitis may also be relieved by a bowel cleanse. Symptoms of abdominal pain, intestinal cramping, diarrhea, constipation, and dysentery as well as disorders of the mouth, teeth, nose and throat, may be indicators of an imbalance here.

- **Emotional Imbalances:** The large intestine meridian is involved with the feelings of sadness, and grief. An imbalance of Ki in the large intestine meridian can result in feeling introverted, depressed, irritable, discouraged, stuck and apathetic. Chronic low self-esteem impairs one's ability to move forward.

- **Peak Hours:** 5 a.m. - 7 a.m.

- **Ascribed Colour:** White/ Silver

- **Location:** This meridian begins at the outside edge of the index finger. It travels up the edge of the finger and then passes between the two tendons of the thumb at the wrist. From there, it moves along the outside edge of the forearm to the elbow. It continues up the arm to the shoulder. It then passes over the shoulder to the shoulder blade, then returns to the muscle at the side of the neck. It runs up the neck and across the cheek. It passes over the top lip and ends beside the nostril.

Transformational Affirmation:

I surrender, eliminate, and release, all that no longer serves my physical, emotional, mental and spiritual well-being.

LARGE INTESTINE - LI

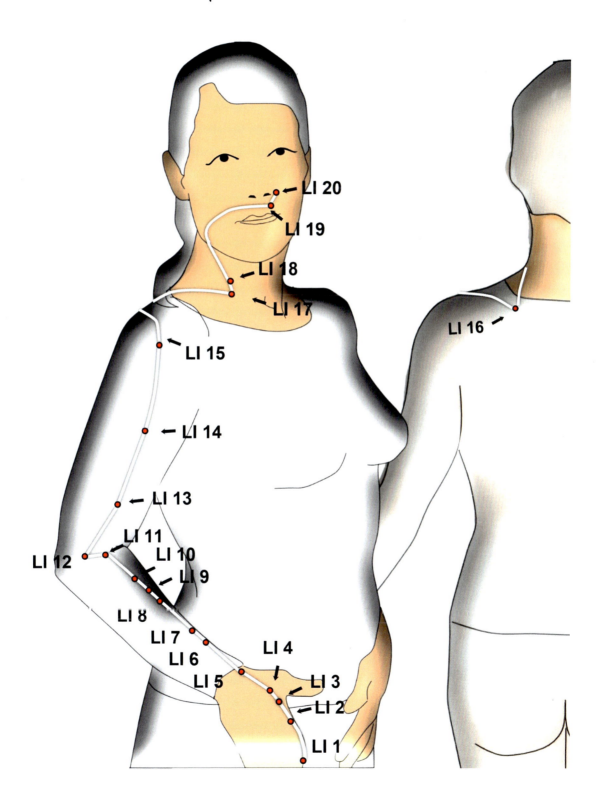

THE GOVERNING VESSEL

The Governing Vessel is known as the *Sea of Yang,* and its energetic flow corresponds to the yang, positive polarity, and masculine aspect. The Yang energy of this meridian governs over all of the yang meridians.

Its complementary channel, is the Conception Vessel, where the energetic flow is yin in nature. Together, they form the Great Central Channel. As such, they are inseparable and facilitate a yin/yang balance throughout the whole body.

The Governing Vessel (Yang) forms the Microcosmic Orbit with the Conception Vessel (Yin).

As we have seen in the Microcosmic Orbit, when Yang Fire merges with Yin Fluid Essence they fuse the Fire and Water Elemental energies together. This fusion facilitates a masculine/feminine balance throughout the body.

- **Physical Imbalances:** An imbalance in the flow of Ki through the governing vessel may result in a range of bodily ailments from a stiff neck to sexual dysfunction, bowel problems, or lower back issues.
- **Emotional Imbalances:** Imbalances in the flow of Ki may show up as lack of insight, clarity, being unrealistic, feeling ungrounded and unloved. Weak willed or unable to stand up for one's self. "Lack of backbone" is the outcome.
- **Location:** The governing vessel begins at the root of the spine, and moves upward through the coccyx and sacrum. It then passes upward through the spine and enters the brain. It passes over the top of the head, over the forehead and then across the bridge of the nose to end at the gum under the top lip. (Internally, this vessel also has branches that link up with the kidneys and heart).

Transformational Affirmation:

I am confident that I am supported and know I can do all that I am called to do.
I am not afraid to take a stand.

GOVERNING VESSEL - GV

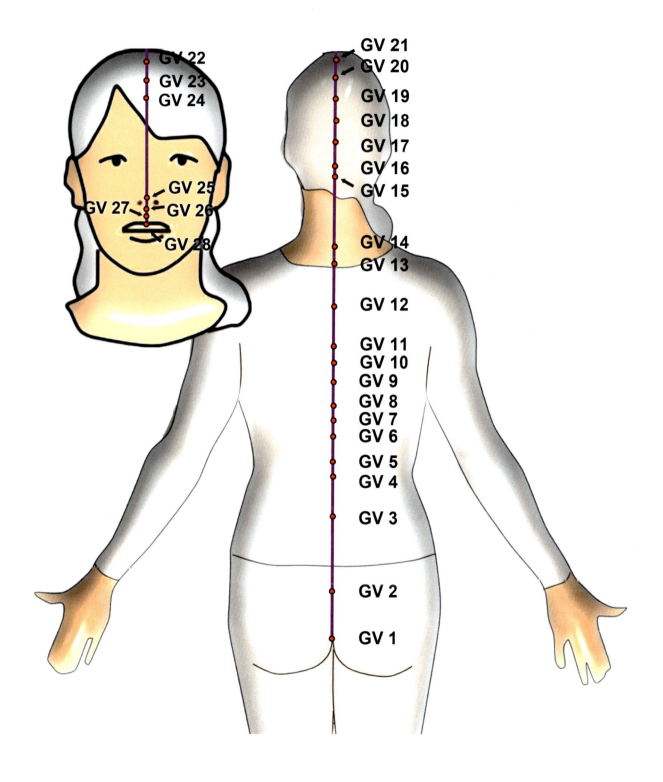

THE CONCEPTION VESSEL MERIDIAN

Known as the *Sea of Yin*, the Conception Vessel, also plays a significant role in the circulation of Ki throughout the body. This vessel is in charge of monitoring and directing all of the Yin channels of the meridian system. The conception vessel forms the circular singularity with the governing vessel in the Microcosmic Orbit.

As we discussed earlier, the Conception and the Governing vessels are considered the most influential among the Ki channels. To effectively balance the flow of Ki in our own bodies, as well as learn to consciously direct and transport it, these are the vessels we must strengthen and train.

**The Conception Vessel (Yin) forms the Microcosmic Orbit
with the Governing Vessel (Yang).**

- **Physical Imbalances:** An imbalance in the flow of Ki through the conception vessel may result in a wide range of bodily ailments These include conditions of the mouth, throat, esophagus, stomach, heart, womb, bladder and sexual organs.

- **Emotional Imbalances:** The front of our body is quite vulnerable. It is soft and open to attack if we compare it to our back. Imbalances in the flow of Ki through the Conception Vessel may manifest as feeling wounded, embarrassed, shy, humiliated, weak, or bullied. These indications are associated with the imprint that the feminine is weaker, the right brain aspirations less valued, etc. If the flow of Ki is weak or imbalanced here, we may feel "less than" and be prone to self-sabotage.

- **Location:** The conception vessel originates at the perineum, and moves upward over the abdomen and chest. It then travels up the centreline of the neck to end just under the lower lip, in the depression above the chin. When the tongue is pressed against the roof of the mouth the bridge between CV 24 and GV 27 is made and the energy of fire and water fuse together in perfect harmony.

Transformational Affirmation:

*I am confident and secure. I remain centred and full of clarity.
There is no challenge that I cannot overcome.*

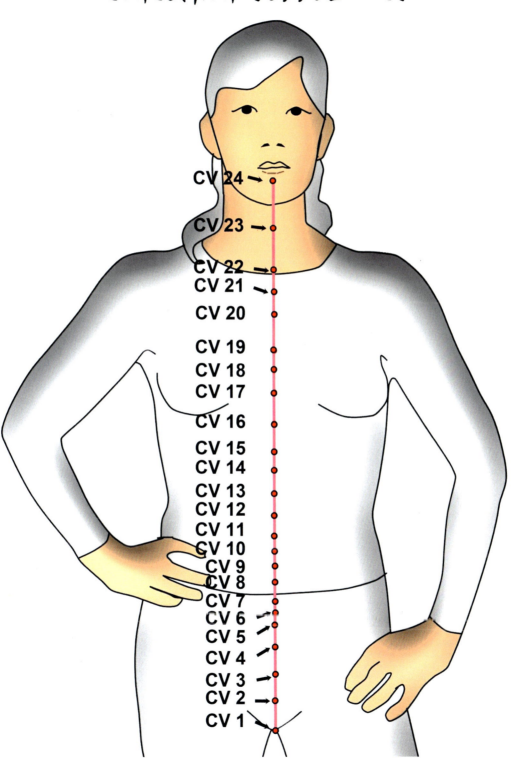

CHAPTER 3

THE FIVE ELEMENTS

For the purpose of Reikiatsu, a basic understanding of The Five Elements will greatly assist you in working with the meridians. When working with the meridians, the premise is, that a person's well-being is dependent on harmony and balance of these five elements.

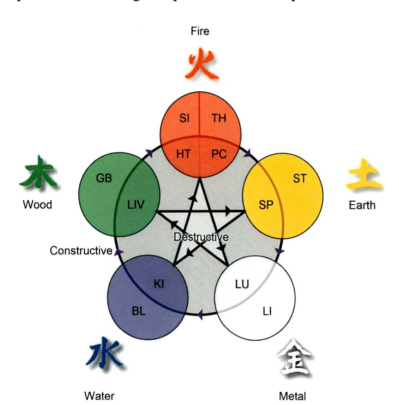

We have seen that all things originate from One Source. Out of this Source, which we call Ki, comes the appearance of Yin and Yang. These masculine/feminine energies then produce the Five Elements. These five aspects are Wood, Fire, Earth, Metal, and Water. These five aspects of Ki are not static, but are always in motion. They also are interdependent, and interact with one another.

The Five Elements participate in the formation of the channels through which Ki flows. These channels connect and nourish all organs and tissues. They also help eliminate toxins out of the body. These Meridians and Five Elements are what we will use in our Reikiatsu Sessions.

THE FIVE GOVERNING ELEMENTS

The five elements govern the form and function of our bodily organs and all aspects of nature. The following are the governing elements of the Yin organs and Yang organs:

Wood: Liver (Yin) - Gall Bladder (Yang)

Fire: Heart (Yin), Small Intestine (Yang), Pericardium (Yin), Triple Heater (Yang)

Earth: Spleen (Yin) - Stomach (Yang)

Metal: Lungs (Yin) - Large Intestines (Yang)

Water: Kidneys (Yin) - Urinary Bladder (Yang)

The Five Element Theory proposes that the two aspects of Ki, which we call Yin and Yang, generate Five Elements that are always in motion and engaging with each other. These dynamic relationships show up as *Constructive or Destructive:*

The Constructive Cycle:

- Wood generates Fire
- Fire generates Earth
- Earth generates Metal
- Metal generates Water
- Water generates Wood

The Destructive Cycle:

- Fire controls or destroys Wood
- Wood controls or consumes Water
- Water controls or destroys (rusts) Metal
- Metal controls or consumes Earth
- Earth controls or smothers Fire

WOOD MERIDIANS: LIVER/GALLBLADDER

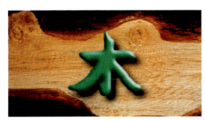

Much like a tree, the wood element can influence our ability to be either rigid or flexible. Our response to life situations sometimes calls for strength and, at other times, for flexibility. The Wood element rules over the emotional and intuitive body. When it is nourished and well balanced, we know when to bend and be flexible and when to stand up and be strong.

Seasonally, Wood Element Ki flourishes in the spring when trees are sprouting new growth. For this reason, the colour of this element is identified as green.

Balanced Wood Element: People who have balanced wood element energy display clarity of mind, personally set goals, and know how to manifest their intentions. They accomplish this by knowing when to persevere and when to yield.

Imbalanced Wood Element: When the wood element Ki is out of balance, a person can be indecisive, without a clear direction in life. They may be defensive and resist when flexibility is required, or give in and yield when they would be better off standing up for themselves.

FIRE MERIDIANS: HEART/SMALL INTESTINE/PERICARDIUM/TRIPLE WARMER

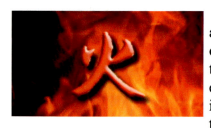

Fire, is the most Yang, or masculine, of the five elements. It is associated with the South, summertime and solar energy. It rules over passion, intensity, desire, intuition, understanding, imagination, and possibilities. Fire both cleanses and purifies. It is considered both constructive and destructive. It may consume everything in its path, or it can offer warmth and cook food. It has the power to transform everything it touches.

The Fire Element's Ki flourishes in summer, the time of heat, growth, warmth, and increased light. This fire is the vibrant red, creative, spark within us all. It promotes courage and strength, helping us to fight for what we want.

Balanced Fire Element: People who have balanced Fire energy may be quite charismatic. They excel at commanding others to action. They may love talking and socializing. A balance in Fire Element energy allows people to become warm-hearted and express love, passion, leadership, spirituality, insight, assertiveness, intuition, and joy.

Imbalanced Fire Element: When the Ki of Fire Element is imbalanced and weak, a person may be dull or boring. They may suffer from frigidity, anxiety, restlessness, and insomnia. They may stammer, talk rapidly, or laugh nervously. A person with an imbalance in the fire element can be too easily stimulated to excess, or they may cold and numb. When the fire element is out of control, a person can become very intimidating and usually pushes people away.

EARTH MERIDIANS: STOMACH/SPLEEN

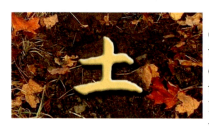

Late summer is the season of the Earth Element. It is associated with Mother Earth and the time of harvest. It assures us that the autumn and winter will pass without difficulty. It speaks to us of how a well-balanced person will do the work it takes during their own spring and summer. This means, that in the fall of their lives they will have the strength of body, clarity of mind, healthy relationships and harvest the abundance of their years.

The Earth Element's Ki thrives in Indian Summer. This is the golden time of abundance before the light diminishes and winter sets in. The colour ascribed to this element is yellow.

Balanced Earth Element: People with fully developed and balanced Earth energy are well-adjusted and grounded. These are empathetic and compassionate people who have an abundance of experience and are willing to share it. They make wonderful counsellors and great friends.

Imbalanced Earth Element: People that have weak or imbalanced Earth Ki are likely to be worriers, exhibit a victim mentality and needy. They will have little compassion for the needs of others but at the same time complain that no one provides for them.

METAL MERIDIANS: LUNG/LARGE INTESTINE *(Sometimes referred to as Spirit Element)*

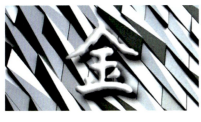

The Metal Element's season is autumn. This is a time where we truly learn more about ourselves. After the harvest of our summer's abundant growth, we are counselled to let go and journey inward as we prepare for a fresh start. Letting go can be a challenge, but unless we are able to release, we surround ourselves with what is in the process of decay and our lives tend to become stagnant and stale.

The Metal Element's Ki peaks in the coolness of autumn. This is a peaceful period for us to discover what is essential, pure and spiritual. The colour of the Metal element is silver/white.

Balanced Metal Element: Someone with well-balanced metal energy is open to the nature of seasonal cycles and the cleansing process of letting go and moving on. Life becomes a continuous adventure of embracing the joyous experience of fresh revelations, and discarding what no longer serves us.

Imbalanced Metal Element: A person with a metal element imbalance will often be overcome with grief over loss, or separation. Saddened by memories of what used to be, their present experiences feel pale in comparison. The will have difficulty growing in new ways and being open to new and vibrant relationships.

WATER MERIDIANS: KIDNEY/BLADDER

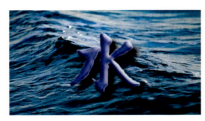

The Water Element is the element of winter and manifests as the power of will, ambition, determination, perseverance, and resolve. These are qualities arising from having a full reservoir of Ki. Winter is a time of quiet repose and hibernation. This is a time where we go within and review. Winter is a period of regeneration, as we conserve ourselves and prepare for new growth in the coming spring.

The Water element Ki rules in the coldness of winter. This is a season when the nights are longer and the darkness prevails. This is a period that asks for patience. The colour of Water element is blue /black.

Balanced Water Element: When the Water Element Ki is strong, a person is courageous and determined. They able to overcome challenges by knowing when to conserve energy and when to direct it towards their goals.

Imbalanced Water Element: When the Water Element Ki is weak and imbalanced, a person will demonstrate a lack of power. They will be insecure and withdraw from projects prematurely. They may be even phobic when it comes to being involved, as they have no sense of personal power.

CHAPTER 4

REIKIATSU SESSIONS

DIRECTING KI INTO THE MERIDIANS

Reikiatsu is a non-invasive way to work with the meridians. It does not rely on hard pressure or the use of implements. In Reikiatsu, Ki is consciously guided through the meridians or a specific point. By building up the Ki in your Hara and drawing it up using the Macrocosmic Orbit, the flow of Ki is transported through the recipient as a dynamic surge of energy. This wave flows into the meridians and brings balance to the yin and yang of their system.

The function of the meridian system is to circulate Ki throughout the body. When the free flow of Ki is interrupted this leads to a lack of energy (Kyo) and an excess of energy (Jitsu).

These blockages may be caused by stress, injury, traumatic experience, or unhealthy habits. Removing these blockages through energetic stimulation or sedation, can balance the human body meridian system, and restore physical, mental and spiritual health.

"Supply energy where there is deficiency and sedate energy when there is an excess."
~ The Yellow Emperor's Classic of Internal Medicine

LETTING YOUR INTUITION GUIDE YOU

Trust your inner guidance system. Begin to direct the energy once the activity in your Hara tells you to. As you were most likely taught in Reiki, your intuition will tell you when enough is enough. Follow your heart.

Consciously direct the Ki flow into or towards the meridian and then beyond into infinity. This way you are not building up energy in the recipient and perhaps causing another imbalance.

By directing Ki to infinity, the flow of energy brings freshness, harmony, and balance to the recipient. It is much like spring rains that restore vitality to a river, as it flows unhindered to its source.

You are supported and you are loved.
As you move out of your way, you freely channel Universal Life Force Energy.
You truly are the Light of the world.

HAND POSITIONS

These are a few hand positions used in transporting Ki with Reikiatsu, that will differ slightly from the way you use your hands with Reiki. These are not the only ways to transport Ki with your hands. You may want to experiment in your practice and find other ways that work for you. The attached pictures should adequately define the suggested positions:

- No Contact Position
- Two Thumb Position
- The Two Finger Position
- The Grip Position
- The Gentle Touch Position

We will look at these briefly now, and later, when we go through the Meridian System, we will come to a greater understanding of their applications.

NO CONTACT TECHNIQUE HAND POSITIONS

This position is one that, as a Reiki practitioner, you are very familiar with. The energy is directed and transported over a distance with no physical contact at all. This may be a matter of inches or hundreds of miles. This energy is consciously directed with the intent that the yin and yang of the recipients meridian system are balanced and restored to perfect harmony.

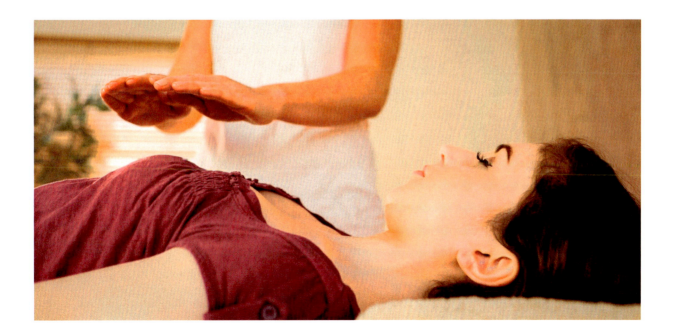

TWO THUMB TECHNIQUE HAND POSITIONS

In this position, the Ki is transported to two points on parallel meridians. The hands may be held in a fist, as in the picture, or open, with the two thumbs applying a gentle pressure to the points.

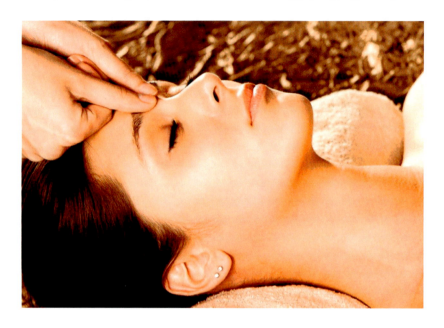

TWO FINGER TECHNIQUE HAND POSITIONS

In this position, the index fingers are placed on the specific points of the left and right meridian that you are currently working with.

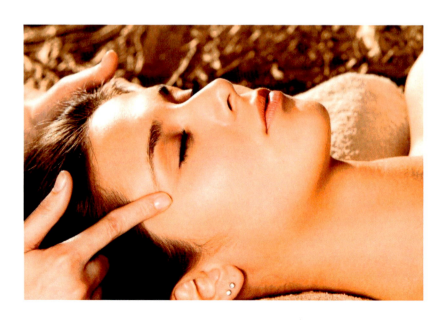

GENTLE TOUCH TECHNIQUE HAND POSITIONS

In this position, the Ki is gently directed through the recipients meridian or point. There is no deep pressure applied. Sometimes, one hand may be focused on a specific point while the other hand remains stationary and supportive. At other times, both hands channel the flow of Ki through parallel meridians.

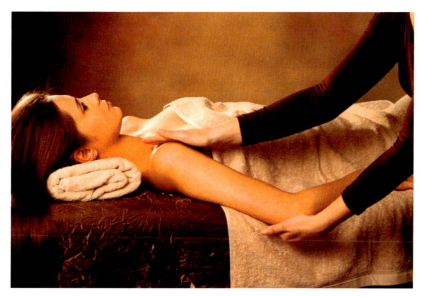

GRIP TECHNIQUE HAND POSITIONS

In this position, there is a slight gentle pressure applied with the open thumb and four fingers of one hand. The other hand may passively support the limb you are working on or simply rest on the limb.

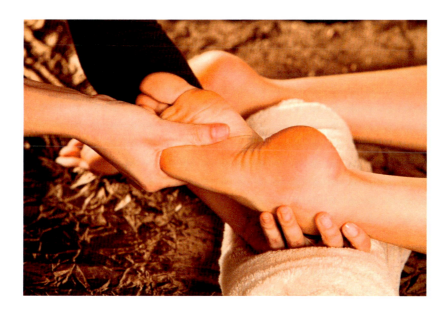

ADDRESSING, SPIRITUAL, EMOTIONAL, AND MENTAL, ENERGY IMBALANCES WITH REIKIATSU SESSIONS

In chapters 2 and 3, we covered some of the imbalances that occur with either an excess or a depletion of Ki in each of the meridians. The Reikiatsu sessions, that will be presented in this chapter, will be focusing on how imbalances of Ki, energetically adversely affect the body's systems physically, spiritually, mentally and emotionally. These imbalances affect our degree of happiness, peace, and vitality, at all levels of being. When the indications of an imbalance are addressed, the physical body responds accordingly, and overall health is the outcome.

The instructions that follow are a guideline. Your intuition will direct you as to the time spent on each pose. You may also be guided to consciously direct the flow of Ki into a specific point. When that is the case, use the hand position and technique that best suits the intention.

Please Note: Unlike Shiatsu or Acupressure, Reikiatsu is primarily dependent on the pressure of the flow of Ki to shift the imbalances, rather than the pressure of the touch. Also take note that the exact location of the points are not as important as the flow of Ki and your intention. These sessions are suggested as a guide, only. How you choose to direct the flow of Ki into the meridians is unlimited.

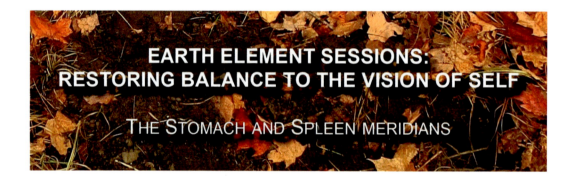

We will begin this section by addressing Earth Element issues that pertain to a lack of groundedness. A person with these indicators expresses their experiences as feeling detached, undernourished, and plagued by a chronic lack of resources.

To move beyond these obstacles, the energy of the Stomach and Spleen meridians, require a balance of yin/yang energy. These are the channels that govern core rooted self-esteem, self-worth, self-value, self-identity, and feelings of empowerment. It is here we develop our origins of feelings. What we "feel in our gut" is reflected back to us by the world around us.

When harmony and balance are achieved in these meridians, one is able to become a calm, compassionate being that is centred and grounded. This enables them to enjoy the support of healthy relationships, and feel abundantly provided for.

EARTH ELEMENT REIKIATSU SESSION - STOMACH MERIDIAN (YANG):

- **Physical Imbalances:** Abdominal cramps, bloating, nausea, vomiting, and sometimes sore throats or halitosis.
- **Emotional Imbalances:** These show up as feelings pertaining to worrying, disappointment, anxiety attacks, insecurity, abandonment, emptiness, lack, distrust, and self-centeredness.

Balancing the Stomach Meridian with a Reikiatsu Session:

By initiating the Macrocosmic Orbit and transporting the flow of Ki into this meridian, any energetic imbalances of the Stomach Meridian will be released. This nourishing flow releases gloom and restores calmness, openness and inner peace. A balanced stomach meridian awakens one's nurturing abilities. This will continue to grow as one finds the rewards that come with helping or validating others.

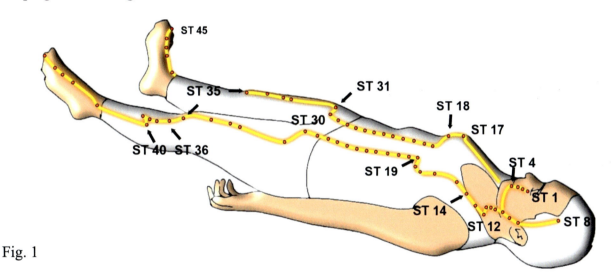

Fig. 1

The Stomach Meridian Reikiatsu Session Procedure:

- In this session begin at the head of the table and engage the Macrocosmic Orbit.
- Start by using the No Contact technique over ST points 1, 2, 3 and 4. This is a similar hand position you use in traditional Reiki. Hover over the points until guided to move on to the next position. Feel the "pressure" of the Ki flow through you as you exhale the Universal Life Force to these meridian points and into the channel.

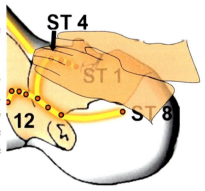

- When guided to move on, place your hands (Gentle Contact) on the jaw line and cover points, ST 5, ST 6, and ST 7. Feel the flow of Ki pass into these points and up the meridian towards ST 8 at the hairline. When you sense it to be clear, lift your hands and move to the next position.

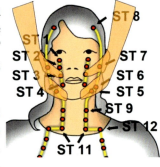

- Now you will use the Two Finger technique on the two ST 8 points, which you can see in the picture are just below the hairline. Trust your intuition, and envision the flow of Ki passing down the channel towards ST 9 (on the throat), and on into infinity. When the flow is clear move on.

- Use both hands in the traditional No Contact position to hover over the throat points, ST 9 to ST 11. Feel the Ki flow through you as you exhale the Universal Life Force through you to these meridian points.

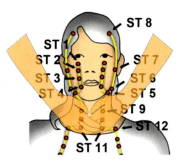

- When flow feels complete, shift to the Gentle Touch technique, placing the thumbs of your hands, on both ST 12 points, (in the depression just under the collarbone). Channel the flow of Ki into both of these parallel points.

- Place your hands in the familiar Gentle Contact position on the ST 13, and ST 14 points. These are on the upper chest below the collar bone. (See Fig 1) Envision the flow.

- No Contact technique is used over the chest points ST 15, through to ST 18. Sense the surge of Ki as it flows through your hands while they hover over these points.

- You will now move to the side of the recipient and, using the Gentle Touch, place your hands on the ST 19 points (below the breasts). Consciously direct the Ki through the parallel channels that pass through the abdomen. Repeat on all abdominal points from ST 20 to ST 27.

- No Contact technique is used as your hands hover over the groin area points, ST 28, ST 29, and ST 30.

- You will now move along side to the recipient's hips and using the Two Finger or Two Thumb technique direct the flow of energy into both of these ST 31 points.

- When guided, shift to using either the Gentle Touch or the Two Thumbs technique, and channel the flow through the leg points from ST 32 through to ST 41.

- On the foot points, ST 42 through to ST 45 (ending on the outside edge of the second toe), apply gentle pressure to the point, using the Grip technique. Your thumb will be placed on the point as you grip the foot. You can either do each foot separately while you support the foot with the other hand, or do both feet simultaneously while channelling Ki through the meridian to infinity.

- End this meridian session holding both ankles and with a finishing exhalation, through the mouth, envision a Cho Ku Rei pass through the entire recipient to infinity.

EARTH ELEMENT REIKIATSU SESSION - THE SPLEEN MERIDIAN (YIN):

- **Physical Imbalances:** Digestive and stomach problems, bloating, flatulence, loose stools and sluggishness.
- **Emotional Imbalances:** Indicators are feelings and experiences such as worry, indifference, hopelessness, poor concentration, forgetfulness, addictions, living vicariously through others, jealousy, self-pity, and low self-esteem.

Balancing the Spleen Meridian a with Reikiatsu Session:

In this session the transported flow of Ki will restore balance and harmony to the energy of the Spleen Meridian. It will awaken and restore openness, introspection, and a rebuilding of self-esteem. Directing Ki into this meridian, will ground and centre the individual, so that they can shift from codependency issues to self-approval and self-control.

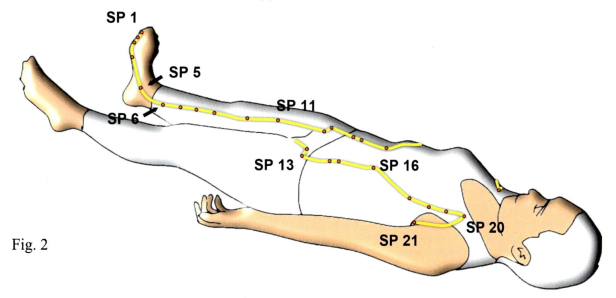

Fig. 2

The Spleen Meridian Reikiatsu Session Procedure:

- Standing at the left hand side of the table, (beside the recipient's left knee) begin the Spleen session at SP 1. You will be using the Grip technique from SP 1 through to SP 9.

- To do this, place your left hand passively on the recipient's left ankle. Using the Grip technique reach across and grasp their right foot with your right hand and gently apply moderate pressure, with your right thumb, on the SP 1 point on the side of the big toe. Activate the Macrocosmic Orbit and envision the flow of Ki passing through the spleen meridian and on to infinity.

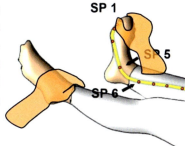

- Continue down the foot and up the right leg, at the meridian points Sp 2 to SP 9. Move ahead to the next point when you feel the flow runs clear.

- When the flow feels clear, move to the right side of the table and reach across with your reach across and grasp their left foot with your left hand, (as you did before with the right), and repeat the procedure to points SP 1 to SP 9 on their left leg. Your right hand will rest passively on their right ankle.

- From either side of the table and using the Grip technique, reach over and grasp the both legs just above the knees with both of your hands. Placing your left thumb on SP 10 (which is two thumb widths above the knee on the inside of the leg). Your right hand will be doing the same technique on the left leg SP 10 point. Channel the flow until clear.

- Using the same technique repeat the procedure on the SP 11 points. (SP 11 is about 7 inches above the SP 10 on the inside thigh). Use your intuition to find these points or use the Gentle Touch and channel Ki into the meridian at this area.

- Using the No Contact technique place your hands hovering over the SP 12 and SP 13 points on both sides of the recipient (See Fig. 2). Feel the flow of Ki passing through you and through the meridian to infinity.

- You may use the Gentle Touch technique on the abdomen points SP 14, SP 15, and SP 16 while channelling Ki through these points. Remember to maintain your breathing while utilizing the Macrocosmic orbit to maximize the flow of energy through your hands.

- On points, SP 17, and SP 18 hover over the chest area using the No Contact technique. Continue to envision the flow of Ki passing through to infinity. You may also exhale and envision the Cho Ku Rei as you direct the energy through your hands.

- Move to the recipient's head for the end of this meridian's session. Gently place your hands on their upper chest area so that the heel of your hands rest on SP 20, your two thumbs can channel Ki into the SP 19 points while your fingers direct energy into the SP 21 points.

- End this session with an invocation of gratitude and with the intention that the Spleen Earth Element Meridian has been cleared and balanced for the recipient's highest good and well being.

Note: Some of these instructions tend to repeat. This is intentional. After a while, these procedures will become second nature to you. Until then, repetition is simply a way to assure you are becoming completely familiar and confident in the methods provided.

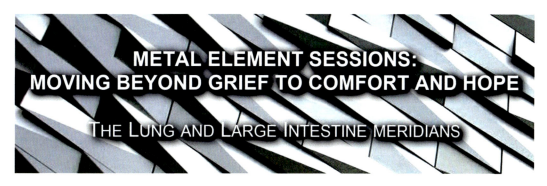

METAL ELEMENT SESSIONS: MOVING BEYOND GRIEF TO COMFORT AND HOPE
THE LUNG AND LARGE INTESTINE MERIDIANS

We now move to those sessions that deal with the ability to let go of the old and accept change and renewal. Imbalances in the Metal Element result in a person persistently hanging on to the past. They are clinging to a nostalgic grief that obstructs change and movement.

To move beyond these obstacles, and move into an experience that is open to the rhythm of the seasons, the highs and the lows, the inhalations and the exhalations, is the experience of a energy system that is balanced. In this state, we welcome the new experiences and cherish the moment. We move beyond grief and a sense of loss, to the comfort of pleasant memories. These are the foundation blocks upon which we build new experiences that fill us with gratitude.

Balanced Ki in the Lung and Large Intestine meridians enable us to become free to breathe. These are the meridians that govern our ability to flourish. When balanced we become a tranquil and inspired being, that is full of spontaneity and childlike freshness.

METAL ELEMENT REIKIATSU SESSION - THE LUNG MERIDIAN (YIN):

- **Physical Imbalances:** Various conditions in the chest, lung, throat and nose. Asthma, sinusitis, allergies, coughing, wheezing, chromic congestion,and the common cold.
- **Emotional Imbalances:** These conditions are expressed as grief, disappointment, despair, anxiety, shame, jealousy,disdain, prejudices, intolerance, and feelings of sadness, and the need to hide or be reclusive.

Balancing the Lung Meridian with a Reikiatsu Session:

Channelling Ki through this meridian will help restore the ability to accept change and process loss in a healthy way. The future will look brighter as the recipient breathes in the new and releases the old. A renewed sense of self-worth, personal integrity, and higher self-esteem comes from a balanced and harmonious lung meridian and strong metal element.

The Lung Meridian Reikiatsu Session Procedure:

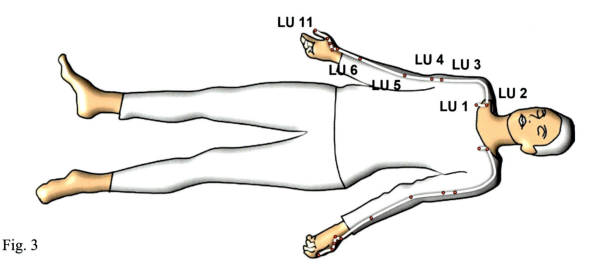

Fig. 3

- Begin the session standing at the head of the table. Using both hands, begin at LU 1 using the Two Thumb technique. Gently apply pressure and direct the flow of Ki to both of the LU 1 points. (About 1 inch below the depression that is under the collar bone). You will consciously direct the flow of Ki through these points of the Lung Meridian. Repeat this procedure on both of the LU 2 points as well, (directly in the depression under the collar bone).

- Move to the left side of the table and cradle the recipient's left hand with your left hand. Using your right hand, place your thumb on LU 3 using the Grip Technique. Your right hand's fingers should be wrapped around their upper arm as you apply pressure with your thumb at the biceps. Consciously direct Ki into the point and through the meridian. Use your Macrocosmic orbit to channel the flow of Ki. Envision the flow passing through the recipient to infinity.

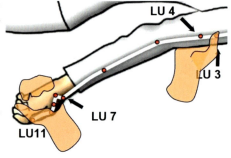

- Maintaining the passive holding position with your left hand, move your right hand down to LU 4 and repeat the same procedure.

- Repeat the above procedure with the Grip Technique on points LU 5, (just inside and below the elbow) and LU 6, on the forearm.

- Continue the same procedure as you apply gentle pressure to points LU 7 through LU 11. Use your right thumb to channel the flow of Ki into the points at the wrist, on the thumb pad, and ending with the LU 11 point at the inside edge of the thumbnail.

- Move to the other side of the table and repeat the procedure moving down the lung meridian points on the recipient's right arm and hand.

- Move to the head of the table. Place both your hands on the recipient's shoulders (Gentle Touch Technique) and channel Reiki through the recipient until you feel completion.
- End the Lung Meridian session with a finishing exhalation, through the mouth. If guided you can visualize a Reiki symbol of your choice pass through the entire recipient to infinity.

METAL ELEMENT REIKIATSU SESSION - THE LARGE INTESTINE MERIDIAN (YANG):

- **Physical Imbalances:** Abdominal pains, cramping, diarrhea, and constipation.
- **Emotional Imbalances:** Disharmony in energy here makes it difficult to let go of prejudices, and intolerance, as well as feelings of sadness, grief, aloofness. disappointment, grief, despair, anxiety, shame and jealousy.

Balancing the Large Intestine Meridian with a Reikiatsu Session:

Consciously directing Ki through the large intestine meridian can help the recipient to function in the world more freely. A person with a balanced energy flow in this meridian will be able to release their need to judge, control and be defensive. They will be able to open to new ideas, embrace what is good for them, and let go of what is not in harmony with their highest good. It is this discernment that contributes to their renewed sense of self-esteem.

The Large Intestine Meridian Reikiatsu Session Procedure:

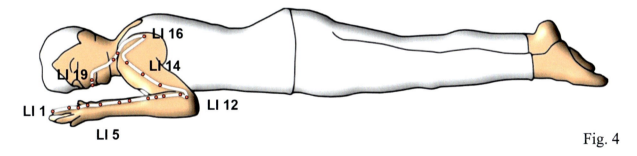

Fig. 4

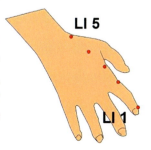

- Engage the flow of Ki through your hands with the Macrocosmic Orbit.
- Move to the recipient's left-hand side and begin this session at LI 1 (on the outside edge of the index finger). You will do this by passively picking up the recipient's left hand with your left hand. Using the Grip technique apply gentle pressure to the LI 1 finger point with the thumb of your right hand. Channel the flow of Ki into the point and the Large Intestine Meridian.

- When the flow feels complete move to the next finger point, LI 2, (inside the index finger at the depression just below the knuckle). Gently apply pressure to the points from LI 1 though to LI 4. Consciously direct Ki flow to and through these points to infinity.

- Continue to to passively support the recipient's left hand. Your active right hand will use the Grip Technique as it applies gentle pressure and consciously directs the flow of Ki into and through points LI 5 to LI 12. You could opt to use the Gentle Touch Technique on these points instead.

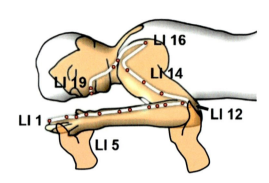

- Feel the "pressure" of the Ki flow through you as you exhale the Universal Life Force through you to these meridian points. Envision the flow of Ki passing through the channel and beyond to infinity.

- When you have completed the flow on point LI 12 , (one thumb width beyond the elbow crease), place the recipient's arm back at rest as depicted in the illustration.

- You may now use the Gentle Touch on points LI 13, through to LI 16. Simply place your hand on their upper arm along the meridian and continue to envision the flow as before.

- When the flow is clear through the meridian to LI 16 you will use the No Contact technique over points LI 17, 18, 19 and 20. Hover over these points at the neck and mouth and channel the Ki generated by the Macrocosmic Orbit. Use your intuition to guide you as to the time spent consciously directing the flow.

- Move to the other side of the table and repeat the sequence on the recipient's right side.

- End this meridian session with both hands resting gently on both LI 16 shoulder points.

- When you feel the session is complete, exhale through the mouth, and envision a Reiki symbol of your choice pass through the entire recipient to infinity.

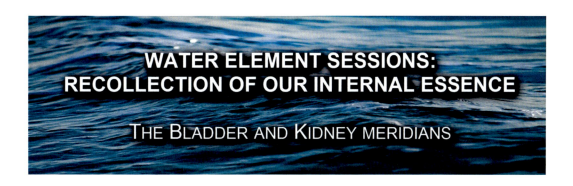

WATER ELEMENT SESSIONS: RECOLLECTION OF OUR INTERNAL ESSENCE

THE BLADDER AND KIDNEY MERIDIANS

We will now consider the Water Element sessions which focus on the fluid and feminine power of rest and motion. Water has the ability to take the path of least resistance and overcome all obstacles in its path. This element is all about remaining true to one's own essence as we navigate through resistance. This element encourages us to go within and reclaim our power. Once we are revitalized we flow freely beyond uncertainty in the knowledge of who we really are.

Balanced Ki in the Bladder and Kidney meridians motivate us to rest as we fill our reserves. It is the recollection of who we really are, that allows us to awaken our innate wisdom and find the courage to flow through life with power.

WATER ELEMENT REIKIATSU SESSION - THE BLADDER MERIDIAN (YANG):

- **Physical Imbalances:** Headaches, backaches, urinary issues and other issues involving bodily fluids. Nosebleeds sometime also occur.
- **Emotional Imbalances:** A person with an imbalanced Bladder Meridian will be feeling indecisive, lethargic, overwhelmed, smothered, empty, uncertain or fearful. Futility, inflexibility and negativity show up as obstacles to making changes.

Balancing the Bladder Meridian with a Reikiatsu Session:

The conscious directing and transporting of Ki through the four spinal branches of the bladder meridian will directly influence the autonomic nervous system and return harmony to the body's basic vital functions. A balanced bladder meridian will revive a sense of determination, will power, and ambition. This session will restore a sense of hope, peace, and tranquility.

The Bladder Meridian Reikiatsu Session Procedure:

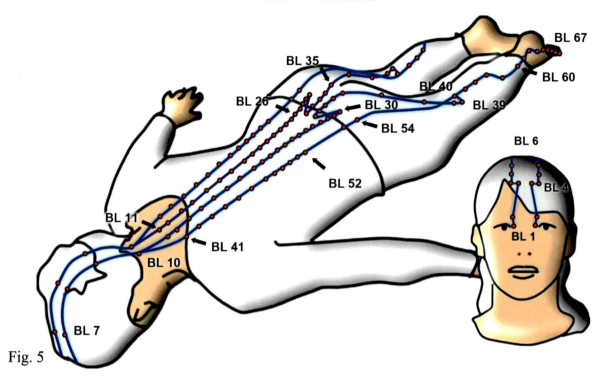

Fig. 5

- Standing at the head of the table initiate the Macrocosmic Orbit and begin this session with the recipient lying on their back.

- (*Another option, if you are doing the Kidney meridian session following the Bladder meridian session, is to do points BL 1 through BL 6 with the Kidney meridian session).*

- Begin at BL 1 using the the Two Finger technique. Apply gentle pressure to both BL 1 face points as you consciously direct energy through them. Continue to channel Ki into and through these points until you are guided to move. Repeat on BL 2 points.

- Use either the Two Thumb or Gentle Touch technique on the the points at the hairline and over the scalp, (BL 3 through to BL 6).

- With the recipient now lying face down we will place both hands on the top of their head and gently use the Gentle Touch technique to channel Ki into the BL 7 points on their crown. Move on to points BL 8 through to points BL 10, when you feel the flow to the set of points is complete.

- Move to the side of the table. Facing the feet, we will now work down the Bladder Meridian points on each side of the spine. Beginning at points BL 11, you will use the Two Thumb or Gentle Touch Technique to channel Ki into the points. Move to the subsequent set of points when your intuition guides you. Envision the flow of Ki passing down the channel as you work through all the points on both sides of the spine from BL 11 to BL 26.

- Using the Gentle Touch Technique, we will now place our hands across the sacrum so that they cover the meridian points, BL 27 to BL 34. Consciously direct Ki into this area and meridian.

- When guided, move down the side of the table so you are beside the recipient's calves and facing the head of the table. Reconnect with the Macrocosmic flow and using the No Contact technique over BL 36 points transport the Ki as before, using your intuition to guide you as to the time spent consciously directing the flow.

- Repeat above procedure using the Two Thumb or Gentle Touch technique to the back of the leg points BL 37, 38, 39 and 40.

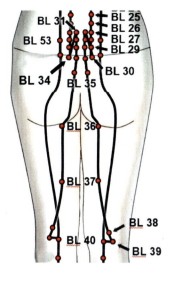

- You will now move back up the side of the table to recipient's shoulder level. The BL 41 to BL 54 points are along the spine four finger widths lateral to both sides of the spine. Engage the Macrocosmic Orbit and channel Ki into these points once again, using the Two Thumb or Gentle Touch Technique. Consciously direct the Ki through the parallel channels on both sides of the body. Move from point to point as you feel guided. (The BL 53 and BL 54 points are 4 finger widths to the outside of the sacrum.)

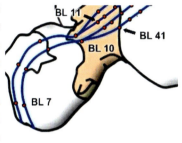

- You will now move down alongside the recipient's calves and using the Two Thumb or Gentle Touch technique, channel the flow through BL 55 to BL 60. Move from point to point as you feel guided while channelling the flow of Ki to infinity.

- Consciously direct Ki into and through the Bladder Meridian using either the Gentle Touch technique or the Two Thumbs technique on points L 61 to BL 67. You can either do each foot separately while you support the foot with the other hand or do both feet simultaneously while channelling Ki through the meridian to infinity.

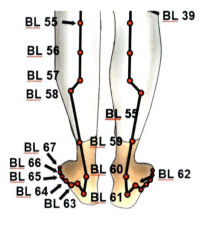

- End this meridian session with hands on the sides of both feet, covering points BL 61 to BL 67. With a finishing exhalation, through the mouth, envision a Reiki symbol of your choice pass through the entire recipient to infinity.

WATER ELEMENT REIKIATSU SESSION - THE KIDNEY MERIDIAN (YIN:

- **Physical Imbalances:** Anemia, chest pains, asthma, abdominal pain, irregular menstruation, or impotence.

- **Emotional Imbalances:** Feelings of fear, paranoia, depression, panic, loneliness, recklessness and insecurity may present themselves as indications of energy imbalances.

Balancing the Kidney Meridian with a Reikiatsu Session: Ki transported into this meridian can restore clarity of mind, self-awareness, present moment appreciation, and a sense of belonging. This renewed feeling of security empowers the individual to express themselves with power yet remain gentle and compassionate.

The Kidney Meridian Reikiatsu Session Procedure:

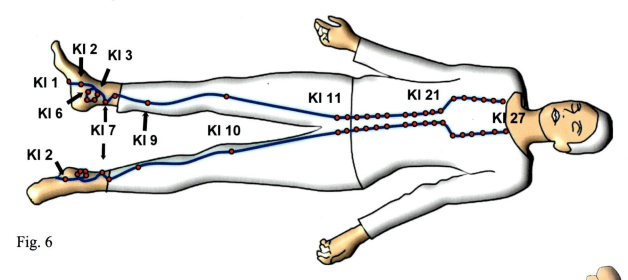

Fig. 6

- Begin the session with the Macrocosmic Orbit. Standing at the foot of the table, use the Grip technique, with your thumbs gently applying pressure to the KI 1 points. Direct the flow of Ki into the points and through the meridian. Visualize it passing through the recipient's body to infinity.

- When you feel it is completely flowing clear, move up to KI 2 points using the same technique. Your hands will be on the tops of their feet with your thumbs on the points as you consciously direct Ki flow to and through these points, as well.

- Place your hands over and use the Gentle Touch technique on points KI 3 to KI 6. These points encircle the ankle bone. Envision the flow of Ki passing through the channel to the head, and beyond to infinity.

- For the KI 7, and KI 8, use the Grip technique, but this time, do one foot at a time. For the recipient's right foot, cradle their heel in your left hand while applying moderate pressure to the point with your right thumb. KI 7 is on the inside border of the Achilles tendon, with K 8 slightly up and forward. Repeat the procedure on the left foot using your opposite hands. Continue to envision the flow as before.

- Move your hands to KI 9 and use the same procedure. KI 9 is 6 inches above the inside ankle bone below the calf. Use the Two Thumbs or Gentle Touch technique.

- Move to the side of the recipient and using the Grip Technique on both legs, consciously direct the Ki through the two KI 10 points with your thumbs on the points. These are just behind the knee joint on the inside depression between the tendons.

- No Contact technique is used as your hands hover over and direct the flow of Ki into the KI 11 and KI 12 points.

- You will now move along side to the hips and using the Gentle Touch technique place your hands on the points KI 13 through KI 16. Channel Ki through these points. Move your hands and again, using the Gentle Touch technique, place them over KI 17 to KI 20, just below the breast. Consciously direct Ki into and through the Kidney meridian.

- No Contact technique is used over points KI 22, an KI 23, as you direct the flow of Ki.

- End this meridian session standing at the head using the Gentle Touch technique on points KI 24 25, 26, and 27. When the flow is clear and you feel guided end with a finishing exhalation, through the mouth, envision a Reiki symbol of your choice pass through the entire recipient to infinity.

Note: It is important to remind you that Reikiatsu is about energy balance and restoring harmony to the system. The exact location is not as critical as it is in acupuncture. Place your hands in the location provided in the illustration and notes, but also feel with your intuition and let it guide you to the spot. You will quickly become very proficient in finding the energy spots that are either Kyo or Jitsu.

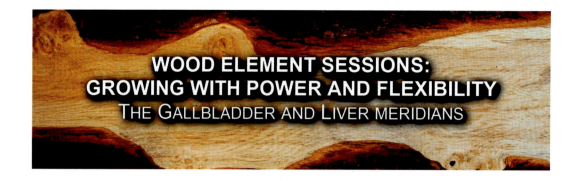

WOOD ELEMENT SESSIONS: GROWING WITH POWER AND FLEXIBILITY
THE GALLBLADDER AND LIVER MERIDIANS

We will now look at the vital sessions that deal with the ability to be decisive. These sessions develop the clarity and wisdom to know when to stand strong and when to bend, when to resist and when to give in. Wood is all about expansion, growth and personal development. Wood branches out and takes risks as it reaches for the heavenly light. At the same time, wood remains well anchored to the earth in the midst of its creative endeavour.

Balanced Ki in the Gallbladder and Liver meridians encourage us to persevere with patience. It is in the delicate dance between reaching for the heavens and remaining true to our stance.

WOOD ELEMENT REIKIATSU SESSION - THE GALLBLADDER MERIDIAN (YANG):

- **Physical Imbalances:** When the Ki flow is weak and this channel is out of balance sleeping patterns are affected. Elimination issues may be a result showing up as bloating, constipation or diarrhea, etc.. Dizziness, may also occur.

- **Emotional Imbalances:** Persons with an imbalance here may be given to various addictions, whether that be addictions to work, sex or substances. These compulsive tendencies may be ways to deal with feelings of resentment, repression, depression, and indecisiveness. A lack of tolerance, anger, arrogance and pretentiousness may mask their inability to respond in a healthy way.

Balancing the Gallbladder Meridian with a Reikiatsu Session: Transporting Ki into this channel can restore courage and initiative, better decision-making skills and judgment. This will lead to undisturbed sleep patterns and the creative, healthy expression of one's goals. Balanced energy here releases the negative inner chatter and toxic thinking that has impaired the clarity and courage required to achieve positive results. It allows us to embrace the higher aspects as we reach upward and yet remain firmly planted in our earthly experiences.

The Gallbladder Meridian Reikiatsu Session Procedure:

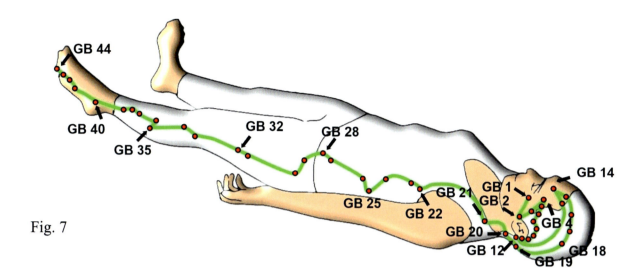

Fig. 7

- Channelling the Macrocosmic Orbit we begin this session at the head of the table. Gently place your two index fingers on both GB 1 points using the Two Finger technique. Consciously direct Ki flow to and through these points.

- Use the Gentle Touch technique Place your hands over the ears. As you exhale, feel the Ki flow through you through the meridian and into points, GB 2 through to GB 12.

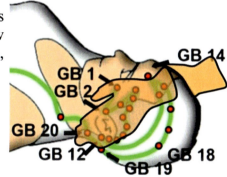

- Using the Gentle Touch technique place your hands parallel over points, GB 14 through GB 18. Continue to envision the flow, of Ki, as before.

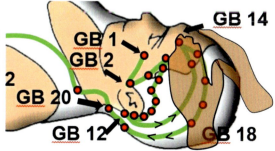

- Once the flow feels completed, gently lift the recipients head and cradle it in your hands. Your fingers should automatically cover the back of the neck points GB 19 and GB 20. Channel the Macrocosmic Orbit and push the Ki through these meridian points as before, using your intuition to guide you as to the time spent consciously directing the flow.

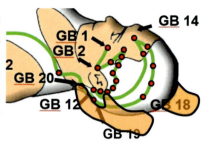

- Using the Gentle Touch, place your hands on the GB 21 points on both shoulders. Engage the flow and direct it through these points into the meridian and beyond. (See Fig. 1)

- Move to the left side of the recipient and consciously direct the Ki through the channels using the No Contact technique hovering over points GB 22 and GB 23.

- Using the Gentle Touch technique, channel the flow through points GB 24 through to GB 30. You may choose to address one point at a time or two points. Simply use your intuition to guide you and everything will clear in the meridian.

- For leg points points GB 31, 32, 33 and 34, use the Two Thumbs technique and apply gentle pressure to the points while you channel the flow of Ki. (See Fig. 7)

- For points GB 35 to GB 44, you may use the Grip or Gentle Touch technique. You will passively hold their left heel with your left hand while you channel the Macrocosmic Orbit Ki flow into the point with your right thumb or hand. Move to the next point when you feel the time is right and repeat. These sessions will finish at GB 44 on the outside edge of the 4th toe.

- When the left side is fully complete move to the other side of the table and repeat the same procedure for points on the recipient's right side.

- End this meridian session with your hands paced on the outside of both feet covering points BL 40 to BL 44. With a finishing exhalation, through the mouth, envision a Reiki symbol of your choice pass through the entire recipient to infinity.

WOOD ELEMENT SESSION - LIVER MERIDIAN (YIN):

- **Physical Imbalances**: Liver meridian imbalance or weakness manifests physically as eye problems and may show up as blurry vision. Brittle fingernails are also a sign of liver meridian Ki imbalance. Hernias, urinary issues such as incontinence may be an issue.

- **Emotional Imbalances**: A person with an imbalance in the liver meridian will have less drive and tend to be weak in ambition. Blockages in energy here can cause irrational anger, and resentment. Negative self-talk and self-loathing are common experiences.

Balancing the Liver Meridian with a Reikiatsu Session: Transportation of Ki throughout this meridian will open the recipient to become more kind and compassionate, especially towards themselves. They will find it easier to let go of resentment and release toxic attitudes. A renewed sense of personal power will make them more able to deal with outside influences that they perceive as negative. This flexibility allows them to grow emotionally out of imprinted habits and behaviours.

The Liver Meridian Reikiatsu Session Procedure:

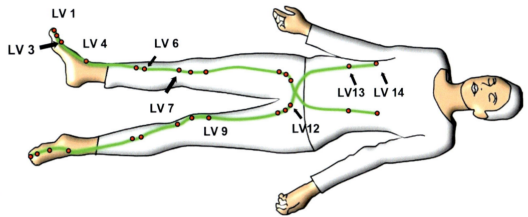

Fig. 8

- At the foot of the table, initiate the Macrocosmic Orbit and begin the session at LV 1, (the inside edges of the big toes) using the the Grip technique. Grasp both feet with your thumbs placed on the points and gently apply pressure as you consciously direct the Ki flow.

- When completed, move your thumbs up to the LV 2 points, and direct the flow of Ki into and through these points. Using the Grip or Gentle Touch technique, repeat the procedure on points, LV 3, 4, 5 and 6. (LV 5 and LV 6 are in the depression at the level of the calf just inside of the tibia).

- Move to the side of the table and, using the Gentle Touch technique, direct the flow of Ki by placing your hands on both of the LV 7 points (just inside and below the knee cap). When this feels complete, move to LV 8 (inside of the knee cap) and continue this procedure. The same technique is applied to LV 9, (just inside and above the knee cap).

- No Contact technique is used over points, LV 10, 11 and 12. These points are along the crease of the leg at the pubic area. Channel the Ki as before, using your intuition to guide you as to the time spent consciously directing the flow.

- Move up the side of the recipient and using the Gentle Touch technique, consciously direct the Ki through the parallel channels just as you would do in Reiki over the abdomen on points from LV 13 and LV 14. (LV 13 is at the bottom of the rib cage on the end of the 11th rib. LV 14 is below the breast).

- End this meridian session with a finishing exhalation, through the mouth, and envision a Reiki symbol of your choice pass through the entire recipient to infinity.

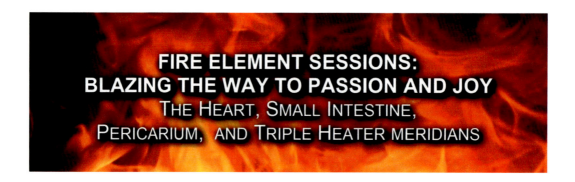

We will now cover the Reikatsu sessions that deal with a person's ability to experience passion, enthusiasm, and joy.

A harmonious balance of Ki in the Fire meridians is required for a person to develop and embody love, passion, intuition, leadership, spirituality, dynamism, assertiveness, logic, and self-expression. The fire personality is fearlessly outgoing. A fire type succeeds by becoming warm-hearted and generous. Expressions of love, compassion, fun, joy, and pleasure are healing experiences for fire individuals.

The **Heart and Small Intestine** meridians are the Fire Element channels that enable us to connect to the loving energies of the heart and express enthusiasm and joy. What we feel in our heart sets the mood for all other emotions. When balanced, we have a powerful and stable platform upon which we can build a healthy and vibrant life. Our love of our self, is equal to the love we have for others.

The **Pericardium and Triple Heater** meridians are the Fire Element channels that, when balanced, allow us to be warm-hearted, stable minded and experience child-like enthusiasm. The Pericardium meridian is also known as the "Heart Protector" as it guards it against the damage the emotions generated by other organs may cause, (Such as anger from the liver, grief from the lungs and fear from the kidneys).

How we love and respect ourselves is ultimately an indication of our ability to love others in a healthy and reciprocal way.

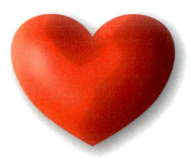

FIRE ELEMENT REIKIATSU SESSION - THE HEART MERIDIAN (YIN):

Physical Imbalances: Shortness of breath, coldness in the chest and limbs, palpitations, cold sweat, inability to speak, memory failure and restless sleep. Arm pains along this meridian may occur.

Emotional Imbalances: The heart is the ruler of all emotions. Signs of imbalance include agitation, sadness, the excess or absence of laughter, depression, fear, anxiety, inconsistent behaviour, loneliness, jealousy, and sorrow. Lack of love for self and broken heartedness are present.

Balancing the Heart Meridian with a Reikiatsu Session:

Consciously directing the flow of Ki through this meridian releases agitated thoughts and connects the person with the loving energies of the heart. When balanced, this meridian will restore tranquility, gentleness, a loving spirit, optimism, a renewed zest for life, and heart-centred wisdom.

The Heart Meridian Reikiatsu Session Procedure:

- Consciously direct the flow through your hands as you channel the Macrocosmic Orbit.

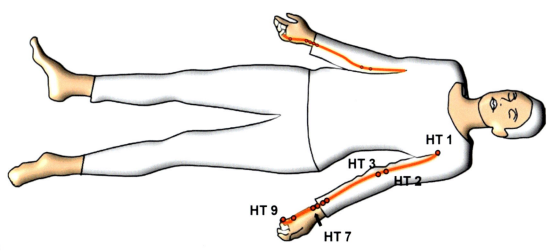

Fig. 9

- Place your left hand in the Grip hand position over the points HT 4, 5 6 and 7, on the recipient's left arm. Allow this hand to remain passive as you use the Grip technique with your right hand to grasp the arm just above the biceps. Place your thumb on the HT 1 point and direct the flow through this point into the meridian.

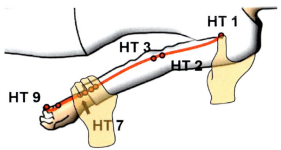

- When the flow feels completed, maintaining the same passive position with your left hand, move your right hand down so that your thumb pressure now is applied to HT 2. Direct the flow of Ki through this point, as well.

- Repeat the above procedure on HT 3 (See Fig. 9).

- When the flow feels clear and completed, allow your right hand to become passive and channel the flow through your left hand into HT 4, 5, 6 and 7 simultaneously. Feel the "pressure" of the Ki flow through you as you exhale the Universal Life Force through you to these meridian points. Envision the flow of Ki passing through your hand, into the meridian and beyond..

- You will now move your right hand down to support the left forearm. Release your left hand from over the above four wrist points and using the Grip technique apply gentle pressure with your thumb to point HT 8. (In the crease just below the knuckle of the little finger). Direct the flow through this point.

- Continue to support the right arm with your right hand and move to the HT 9 point, (inside the little finger beside the fingernail). Send Ki through this point with your intention that the meridian be cleared (See Fig. 9)..

- Move to the other side of the table. Repeat the whole procedure from HT 1 through HT 9 on the recipient's right side.

- End this meridian session with a finishing exhalation, through the mouth, envision a Cho Ku Rei symbol passing through the entire recipient to infinity.

FIRE ELEMENT REIKIATSU SESSION - THE SMALL INTESTINE MERIDIAN (YANG):

- **Physical Imbalances:** Signs include digestive and elimination problems such as abdominal pain, constipation, diarrhea, too much, or too little urination, as well as hearing issues, including tinnitus. A stiff neck may also be an indication.

- **Emotional Imbalances:** A lack of mental clarity that manifests as an inability to evaluate or assimilate ideas. It also shows up as insecurity, a fear of commitment, vulnerability, cynical thinking or sarcasm. A lack of enthusiasm and chronic fatigue is common.

Balancing the Small Intestine Meridian with a Reikiatsu Session:

Channelling the flow of Ki through this meridian assists a person to be happy, lively, and passionate. With a renewed capacity for intimacy, this warm and attractive personality will be filled with a zest for life. Their clarity of mind allows them to achieve much, yet still, find time for quiet introspection.

The Small Intestine Meridian Reikiatsu Session Procedure:

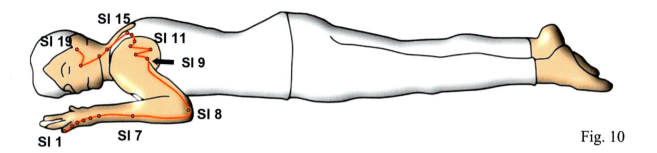

Fig. 10

- Begin this session at the left side of the table. Place your right hand over points S1 to SI 6. Using the Gentle Touch technique channel the flow of Ki into all six points from the little finger to the wrist of the left hand. (Alternatively, you may use the Grip technique and channel Ki into each of the points individually).

- When the flow is complete through SI 6, move your right hand and apply pressure to SI 7 using the Grip or Gentle Touch technique. Consciously direct Ki flow to and through this point to infinity.

- Again, when the flow is complete, move your right hand and apply pressure with your right thumb to the SI 8 elbow point, (it is in the depression between the elbow and the tip of your forearm). Feel the flow of Ki passing up the channel on the arm, and beyond.

- Move to position yourself beside the recipient's elbow. Now place your left hand passively over their elbow point SI 8 and your right hand over the seven shoulder points, SI 9 through to SI 15. Using the Gentle Touch technique channel the flow of Ki through your right hand to these all of these points. Continue to envision the flow as before.

- Raising both hands, use the No Contact technique and hover over four neck and cheek points, SI 16 through SI 19, channel the Ki as before. Use your intuition to guide you as to the time spent consciously directing the flow.

- End this meridian session here when complete, and with a finishing exhalation, through the mouth, envision a Reiki symbol of your choice pass through the entire recipient to infinity.

FIRE ELEMENT REIKIATSU SESSION - THE PERICARDIUM MERIDIAN (YIN):

- **Physical Imbalances**: When the Ki of the pericardium meridian is out of balance a person may experience various disorders of the chest area, including chest pain, heart palpitations, angina, or anxiety attacks.

- **Emotional Imbalances:** An imbalanced pericardium meridian will show up emotionally as feelings of exhaustion, abandonment, depression, invisibility, sexual deviancies, or frigidity.

Balancing the Pericardium Meridian with a Reikiatsu Session:

Consciously directing the flow of Ki through the "Heart Protector" opens the heart to trust again and be filled with joy, and love. This reclaimed discernment awakens us to the potential of warm, intimate relationships, that are fulfilling on all levels.

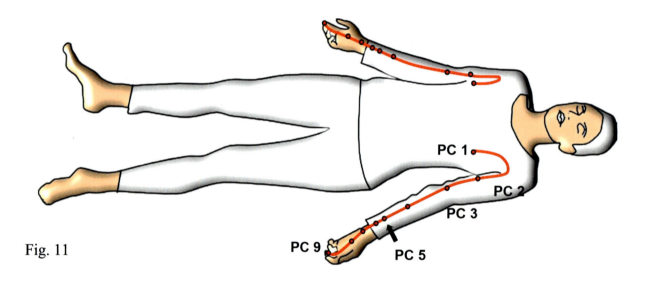

Fig. 11

- Engage the flow of Ki through your hands as you channel the Macrocosmic Orbit.

- Standing beside the recipient's left arm direct the flow of Ki, through your hands, hovering over PC 1 (above the nipple), using the No Contact technique.

- When the flow feels free and unobstructed, place your left hand passively over the recipient's left wrist. Using the Grip technique with your right hand, apply gentle pressure to PC 2 on the inside of their upper left arm between the two folds of the biceps.

- Repeat the above procedure to the points, PC 3, (inside at the elbow joint) and at PC 4.

- Move your left hand from its passive wrist position to pick up and cradle the recipient's left hand. Using the Grip technique with your right hand apply pressure with your right thumb to point PC 5. Feel the flow pass through this point as you channel the Macrocosmic Orbit into and through this meridian.

- Repeat the above procedure to the points PC 6, 7, 8, and finish with PC 9 (at the centre tip of the middle finger). Hold the position until the flow feels clear and complete.

- End this meridian session with a finishing exhalation, through the mouth, envision a Cho Ku Rei symbol passing through the entire recipient to infinity.

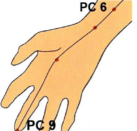

FIRE ELEMENT REIKIATSU SESSION - THE TRIPLE HEATER MERIDIAN (YANG):

- **Physical Imbalances:** Imbalances in the Ki flowing through this meridian may result in headaches, especially in the temples, as well as ear issues. An imbalance in the Ki of this meridian can also show up as feeling flushed, fevers, chills, hot flashes and night sweats. Since an imbalance in the Ki of the Triple Heater meridian "drains" energy from the other meridians it can also contribute to immune disorders, stress, or chronic fatigue.

- **Emotional Imbalances:** These show up as feelings of being overwhelmed, with chronic fight /flight / or freeze impulses occurring. An over-active Triple Heater meridian can cause anxiety, hyper-vigilance, or an over-all exhaustion.

Balancing the Triple Heater Meridian with a Reikiatsu Session: When Ki flows balanced through the Triple Heater meridian a person feels safe, secure and capable of handling all of life's situations. A kind-hearted, stable minded and joyful person now able to break habitual behavioural patterns and evolve to a higher perspective. When the heart beats pure and free of remorse, one is able to live comfortably at peace.

The Triple Heater Meridian Reikiatsu Session Procedure:

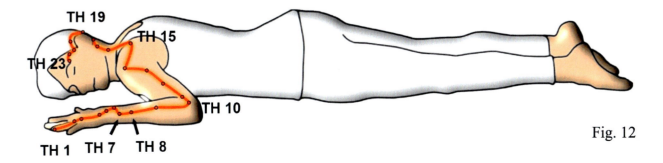

Fig. 12

- Begin the session at TH 1 using the the Gentle Touch technique. Standing at the side of the table near the recipient's head place your left hand over their left hand. Your palm will rest on the recipient's fingers with your middle finger sitting over their hand from their knuckle to their wrist. Simultaneously, direct the flow of Ki into the hand points TH 1, 2 and 3. Channel the Ki until the flow feels complete.

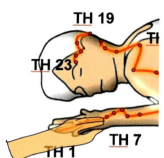

- Now using the Gentle Touch move your left hand and place it completely over the recipient's left wrist points, TH 4, 5 6 and 7. Feel the Ki flow through your left hand into all of these meridian points.

- Allow this hand to become passive as you use the Gentle Touch technique with your right hand on TH 8. Place your right hand over this point and direct the flow into the meridian.

- Your left hand remains passive at the wrist position while you move your right hand over the TH 9 point. Channel the flow of Ki though the point to infinity.

- Repeat the above procedure on points TH 10 through to TH 14. Envision the flow of Ki passing through the channel to infinity. (See Fig. 12)

- When the flow is clear and you feel it is complete, move your right hand into the Gentle Touch technique position over TH 15, and direct the flow into the meridian and point as before.

- Lift your left hand from the passive wrist position and place it hovering over the head points TH 19, 20, 21, 22 and 23. Your right hand will be over the neck points TH 16, 17 and 18. Channel the flow of Ki with this gentle touch technique into these points and through the meridian, using your intuition to guide you as to the time spent consciously directing the flow.

- Move to the other side of the recipient and repeat the procedure on their right hand side. Begin with their right hand and work up the the head points as before.

- End this meridian session with a finishing exhalation, through the mouth, envision a Reiki symbol of your choice pass through the entire recipient to infinity.

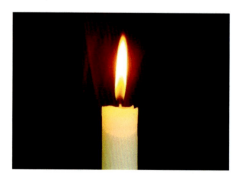

THE THREE TREASURES - THE WISDOM OF TAOISTS SAGES

Before we begin the *Merging River Sessions* of the Governing and Conception Vessels, it seems a good time to reflect on the Three Treasures of Traditional Chinese Medicine.

The Taoist Sages share their wisdom in the form of a metaphor. They say we are similar to a candle. According to them there are three aspects to a candle.

- **Jing:** The wax and wick of the candle, correspond to your physical essence. The material substances that you are composed of are comprised of very condensed dynamic energy. This is the basic root energy that you are made of, and it is called Jing. This Jing essence, allows us to exist on this plane of existence.

- **Chi (Ki):** We then consider, the flame of the candle. This corresponds to your life force energy. Ki is the *breath of life of Source* that empowers you. It is the moving, transformational power that permeates your body and activates it. Entering your body through your nose and mouth it circulates through the meridians to nourish and maintain every part of your being.

- **Shen:** Then there is the radiance of the candle, which corresponds to your spirit. This is the brightness that shines in your eyes. It is the glow that surrounds you as you share your light with the world. Shen is not a feeling. Shen is all-embracing, unconditional Love that resides at your very core. This Divine Spark radiates outward from your heart. Its pure purpose is to express love, kindness, compassion, generosity, giving, tolerance, forgiveness, mercy, tenderness and the appreciation of beauty. It is who "you" really are.

What is important about this knowledge is that when we do the Microcosmic Orbit, we are intentionally involved in the movement and development of these energies.

Normally, your substantial energetic essence called Jing can flow either way through the energy pathways in the body. In the Microcosmic Orbit, Jing is induced through intention, to combine with the Ki as it flows up the Governor vessel during inhalation and then down the Conception vessel upon the exhalation.

For the radiance of your Shen to exist, your Jing and Ki must combine. The material essence that you are, (Jing) and the life breath that activates you (Ki) must combine, for you to shine in your absolute glory.

When Jing and Ki are in balance, the mind is strong, the emotions are under control, and the body is strong and healthy. By combining the flow of Jing and Ki we balance, develop and increase their energies. When their energies increase, we emanate the light of Spirit. (Shen)

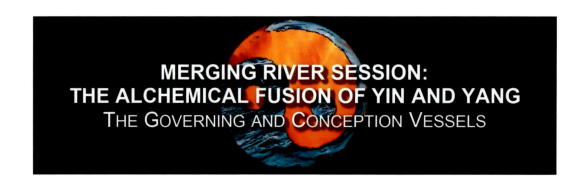

MERGING RIVER SESSION: THE ALCHEMICAL FUSION OF YIN AND YANG
The Governing and Conception Vessels

"The Conception vessel and the Governing vessel are like midnight and midday, they are the polar axis of the body. There is one source and two branches, one goes to the front and the other to the back of the body ... When we try to divide these, we see that yin and yang are inseparable. When we try to see them as one, we see that it is an indivisible whole." ~ Li Shi-Zhen

The Sea of Yang and the Sea of Yin come together to form a powerful central energy loop that all other meridians flow into it like tributaries. It is this alchemical fusion of Yin and Yang energy that nourishes the entire meridian system. When the energies of masculine fire and feminine fluidity merge, the Light of Life is generated.

MERGING RIVER SESSION - GOVERNING VESSEL: (THE SEA OF YANG)

The Governing Vessel Meridian is Yang in nature and begins at the root of the spine. It moves upward through the coccyx and sacrum. It then passes upward through the spine and enters the brain. It passes over the top of the head, over the forehead, and the across the bridge of the nose to end at the gum under the top lip.

- **Physical Imbalances:** An imbalance in the flow of Ki through the governing vessel may result in a wide range of bodily ailments from a stiff neck to sexual dysfunction, bowel problems, or lower back issues.

- **Emotional Imbalances:** Imbalances in the flow of Ki here, may show up as lack of insight, clarity, being unrealistic, feeling ungrounded and unloved. The inability to "stand tall and show some backbone", are consistent with a disharmony here. On the other end of the spectrum, an excess of Ki here may be expressed as a sense of superiority and arrogance.

Balancing the Governing Vessel with a Reikiatsu Session:

When the flow of Yang Ki is balanced and flowing through the Governing Vessel with power, this central Pillar of Light is upright and strong, and the whole meridian system's integrity is maintained. This session will stimulate the flow of Ki to flow through the Governing Vessel, and merge with the Yin energies of the Conception vessel.

When the Ki flow is clear and pure in the Governing Vessel, a person will be confident that they can stand up to any challenge. Directing the flow of infinite Ki into, and through, the governing vessel meridian will facilitate restoration of the yin/yang balance of energy in the body. The recipient will find it easier to let go of notions of superiority or inferiority. A sense of interconnectedness will be re-established as well as a spiritual and physical support.

The Merging Rivers Reikiatsu Session Procedure - Part 1, The Governing Vessel:

(Face down part of the session)

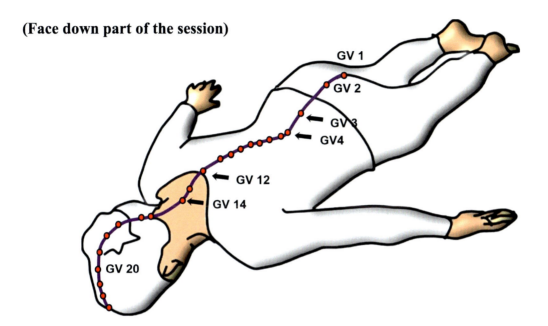

Fig. 13

- Standing at the left side of the table, initiate the flow of Ki, through your hands, with the Macrocosmic Orbit.

- Begin the session at GV 1 using the No Contact technique. Your hands will hover over GV 1 and GV 2, at the base of the spine. Consciously direct Ki flow to and through these points and "push" the flow up the channel towards the crown of the head. Envision the flow travelling through the crown to infinity. Stay here for a while until you feel that the flow is clear and unobstructed.

- Remaining over GV 1 and GV 2, repeat the above but this time it will be a little different. This time envision the flow of Ki passing up the channel to the crown, and see it looping over the top of the head, down the front of their body and returning to your hands. See it as one continuous orbit of fire and water flowing together.

- Place your left hand with the Gentle Touch on GV 14, (where the neck meets the shoulders). Using the Gentle Touch technique, place your right hand on GV 3, (level with the hips). Continue to envision the flow as before, moving beneath your hands, up the spine, over the head, and back down the front, between their legs, to return to your hands.

- Left hand remains on GV 14 as you move to reposition your right hand on GV 4 and repeat the above procedure. Use your intuition to guide you as to the time spent consciously directing the flow (See Fig. 13).

- Repeat directing the flow upwards through the Governing Vessel through points GV 5, to GV 12. You may do this by doing them all at once or by moving your right hand onto the points individually.

- When your right hand is over GV 12 allow it to become the passive hand and channel the Macrocosmic Orbit through GV points 13 and 14 with your left hand. Intend the flow to travel up the channel and over the crown to continue the Merging Rivers loop.

- When your intuition guides you, then you will place your left hand passively on the recipient's left shoulder. Your right hand (Gentle Touch) will be placed over the back of the recipient's head directly over the channel and GV points 15 to 20. The heel of your palm should be on GV 15 at the base of the skull. Stimulate the direction of flow up the channel through points GV 15 to GV 20. Envision the continuous loop flowing over the top of their head and down the front of their body (See Fig. 13).

- This will end the face down part of the session. When the flow is clear and complete remove your hands and when ready ask the recipient to turn over onto their back.

This is, essentially, a Microcosmic Orbit induction.

(Face up part of the session)

- With the recipient now comfortably lying on their back, move to the head of the table. Place your left hand passively on the recipient's left shoulder. Your right hand (Gentle Touch) will be placed over the top of the recipient's head directly over the channel and GV points 21 to 24. Channel the flow through your right hand to GV 24 at the tip of your left hand's middle finger, (in the centre of the forehead, just above the hairline).

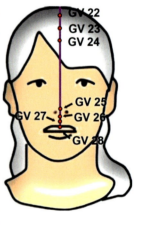

- When the flow feels complete and clear, place your right hand into the No Contact technique over the recipient's nose and mouth. Consciously direct the flow of Ki to GV points 25, 26, 27 and 28. Direct the energy down the Governing Vessel 27/28 to meet the Conception Vessel (at GV 24 just below the lip) and on down the front centreline of the body to the perineum

- End this meridian session in the No Contact technique over these points, and with a finishing exhalation, through the mouth, envision a Reiki symbol of your choice pass through the entire recipient to infinity.

MERGING RIVER SESSION - CONCEPTION VESSEL: (THE SEA OF YIN)

The Conception Vessel Meridian is Yin in nature and originates at the perineum. It normally, travels *upward* over the abdomen and chest, up the midline of the neck to end under the lower lip in the midline, in the depression above the chin. However, when the Sea of Yin is induced through intention to merge with the Sea of Yang it flows *down* the centreline of the body to form a dynamic loop of vital energy that nourishes the whole being.

- **Physical Imbalances:** An imbalance in the flow of Ki through the conception vessel may result in a wide range of bodily ailments These include conditions of the mouth, throat, oesophagus, stomach, heart, womb, bladder and sexual organs.

- **Emotional Imbalances:** The front of our body is the most vulnerable. It is soft and open to attack compared to our back. Imbalances in the flow of Ki through the conception vessel may appear as feeling wounded, embarrassed, shy, humiliated, weak, or bullied. It is associated with the imprint that the feminine is weaker, the right brain aspirations less valued, etc.. If the flow of Ki is weak or imbalanced here, we may feel less than, and be prone to self-sabotage.

Balancing the Conception Vessel with a Reikiatsu Session: When the conception vessel is flowing with Yin energy we feel confident and protected. Consciously directing Ki through this channel will assist the recipient to open up without fear. This will allow them to feel warm and safe without crossing their arms. They will experience a renewed sense of autonomy, and a sovereign right to be heard. They will be able to relinquish their old beliefs regarding being less than worthy, or undeserving, of love and healthy relationships.

The Merging Rivers Reikiatsu Session Procedure - Part 2, The Conception Vessel:

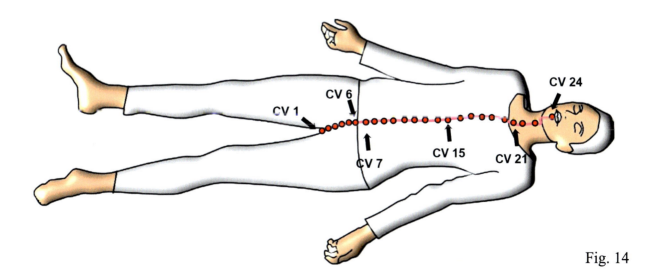

Fig. 14

- This Reikiatsu session follows, sequentially, after the Governing Vessel session. Since we are initiating the continuous loop of Ki, we will begin at CV 24. Your left hand will still rest passively on the recipient's left shoulder with your right hand hovering over CV 24.

- Consciously direct Ki flow to and through CV 24 and envision it flowing down the centreline of the recipient's body. Feel the Ki travel through your hand and pass the full length of their body and loop up the centreline of their back to pass over the top of their head in an infinite unobstructed orbit. (See Fig 14)

- With your left hand remaining passively on their left shoulder, use the No Contact technique to hover over points, CV 23, 22, 21, and 20. Feel the Ki flow through you as you exhale the Universal Life Force through you to these meridian points. Envision the flow of Ki passing down the channel and continually looping as before. When the flow is complete and clear you can move on to the next set of points.

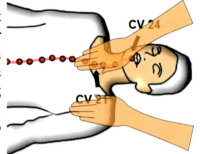

- Place your right hand passively on the recipient's forehead. Using either the No Contact or Gentle Touch technique place your left hand on or over the heart chakra and points, CV 19 through to CV 16. Continue to envision the flow as before. Consciously direct the flow of Ki down the channel in its infinite loop.

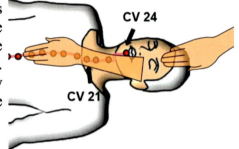

- When you feel the flow is sufficient, move to the side of the recipient place your hands beside each other on the abdomen just below the breast, (Gentle Touch), just as you would do in Reiki. Consciously direct the Ki through the channel, and points CV 15 to CV 7. Remain until your intuition guides you to move on.

- No Contact technique is used as your hands hover over CV 6 to CV 1. Consciously direct Ki into and through the Conception Vessel in its infinite loop ands it merges with the Governing Vessel and travels up the centreline of the back.

- End the Merging Rivers Session with your hands on both feet. With a finishing exhalation through the mouth, envision a Reiki symbol of your choice pass through the entire recipient to infinity.

CHAPTER 5

SPECIFIC POINT - REIKIATSU SESSIONS

WORKING WITH SPECIFIC POINTS TO ACHIEVE EMOTIONAL WELL-BEING

So far, we have focused on Reikiatsu sessions that consciously direct Ki through each of the meridians. The aim is to achieve balance and harmony of Yin and Yang energies in the system.

We will now cover some specific and significant points that can powerfully address emotional issues. Directing Ki into these points can be used to enhance the previous Elemental Reikatsu Sessions or can be used on their own.

STOMACH 36 - 3 MILE POINT - Releasing worry

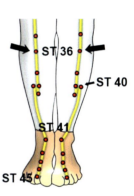

Location: This vital point is found four finger widths down from the bottom of your knee cap, on the outer edge of your shin bone.

Session: Using the Grip technique apply slight pressure with your thumb to the point. Direct the flow of Ki through the point to infinity.

Effects: Restoring the flow of balanced Ki to this point should increase endurance and energy. The balanced earth element returns both stability and grounding. Transmutes the effects of excessive worrying and thinking.

STOMACH 25 - HEAVEN'S PIVOT - Restoring calmness

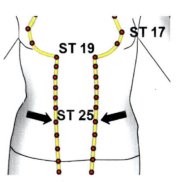

Location: This vital point is found three finger widths on each side of the navel.

Session: Using the Two Thumb technique apply slight pressure with your thumbs to these points. Direct the flow of Ki into these points to infinity.

Effects: Restoring the flow of balanced Ki to this point should calm the mind and sedate the emotions.

SPLEEN 4 - GRANDFATHER GRANDSON - Restoring Self-confidence

Location: This point is found in the depression that is inside and below the bone that follows the big toe.

Session: Using the Two Thumb or Grip technique apply slight pressure with your thumb to the points. Direct the flow of Ki into these points as before.

Effects: Restoring the flow of balanced Ki to this point should reduce the recipient's hyper-excitability, panic attacks, anxiety, nervousness, and restore a sense of self-confidence.

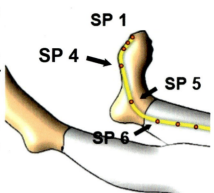

SPLEEN 6 - THREE YIN INTERSECTION - Freedom from toxic emotions

Location: This point is located on the inside of the leg, four finger widths above the highest point of the ankle.

Session: Using the Grip technique apply slight pressure with your thumb to the points. Direct the flow of Ki into these points as before.

Effects: Balancing the energy here pacifies fear, anger, and needless worry. These emotions are the main obstacle to living a happy and fulfilling life.

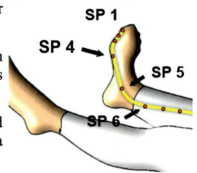

BLADDER 52 - WILL CHAMBER - Uplifting the spirit

Location: This point is located on the back, level with the navel, four finger widths out from the spine.

Session: Using the Two Thumb technique apply slight pressure with your thumb to both of the points. Direct the flow of Ki into these points until guided to release.

Effects: Bringing balance to the BL 52 benefits transformation both mentally and spiritually. Relieving depression and mental exhaustion allows the recipient to move on and find out who they are without these distractions. They get in touch with their inner wisdom and power.

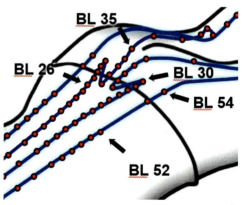

GALLBLADDER 21 - SHOULDER WELL - Expressing emotions

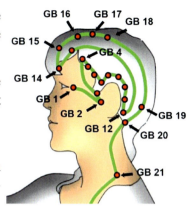

Location: This point is located at the highest point of the shoulder, halfway between the outside tip of the shoulder and the centreline of the back of the head.

Session: Using the Two Thumb technique apply slight pressure with your thumb to both of the points. Use the Sei Hei Ki and direct the flow of Ki into these points until guided to release.

Effects: Consciously directing Ki into and through the GB 21 relieves stress, has a calming effect on the mind. It also assists in the recipient learning to release and express stagnant, buried emotions.

GALLBLADDER 34 - YANG MOUND SPRING - Inner peace

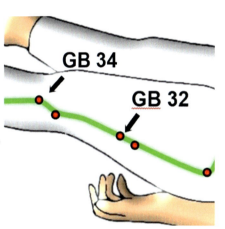

Location: This point is located one and a half finger widths down on the outside of leg below the knee. It is in the depression below the head of the fibula.

Session: Using the Grip technique apply slight pressure with your thumbs to both GB 34 points. Channel the flow of Ki into these points until guided to release.

Effects: Bringing harmony to the Yin and Yang energies of this meridian at the GB 34 point, helps those who are shy and unsure of themselves. It brings flow to those stagnant emotions such as depression, confusion, and irritability and allows the person to become more adaptable and comfortable with situations that previously aggravated them.

GALLBLADDER 44 - YIN PORTALS OF THE FOOT - Resolution of anger

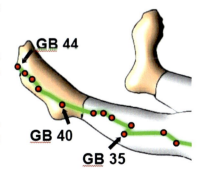

Location: This point is located on the outside of the fourth toe beside the toenail.

Session: Using the Grip technique apply slight pressure with your thumbs to both GB 44 points. Channel the flow of Ki into these points until guided to release.

Transporting Ki into and through the GB 44 facilitates clarity, decisiveness and the ability to focus. Balance the energy here assists in the resolution of anger, frustration, and shyness.

LIVER 1 - GREAT ESTEEM - Increasing self-esteem

Location: On the big toe, at the bottom corner of the nail next to the second toe.

Session: Using the Grip technique apply slight pressure with your thumb to the LV 1 point. Transport the flow of Ki into this point. When you feel guided, repeat procedure on the other toe.

Effects: Balancing the meridian energy through this point enhances discernment around when it is a good time to assert one's self and when it is good to stand down. Knowing what is good for them increases their Self-esteem.

LIVER 2 - MOVING BETWEEN - Expressing emotions in a healthy way

Location: On the foot, in the web between the bones of the big toe and the second toe. It is about half a thumb width above the junction of the two toes.

Session: Using the Grip technique apply slight pressure with your thumbs to both of the LV 2 points. Channel the balanced flow of Ki into these points until you feel guided to release.

Effects: This is a powerful point to release any anger that has been repressed, or expressed in unhealthy ways.

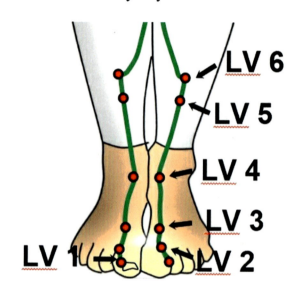

LIVER 3 - GREAT RUSHING - Embracing serenity

Location: On the foot, in the depression between the bones of the big toe and the second toe. It is about 2 finger widths above the junction of the two toes.

Session: Using the Grip technique apply slight pressure with your thumbs to both of the LV 3 points. Exhale the flow of Ki into these points until you feel guided to release.

Effects: This is a powerful point to release blocked emotions and alleviate depression. This point promotes relaxation and serenity.

LUNG 1- CENTRAL TREASURY - Letting go of grief

Location: This point is 3 finger widths below the collarbone. in a depression close to the arm's deltoid muscle.

Session: Using the Two Thumb or Gentle Touch technique, apply slight pressure with your thumb the LU 1 point. Allow the flow of Ki to be pushed through the point and beyond to infinity.

Effects: This point is a key point for initiating the letting go process. Whether someone is grieving the loss of a loved one or something they felt attached to, grieving is natural. This point permits the sense of loss to be dealt with in a healthy and non-overwhelming way.

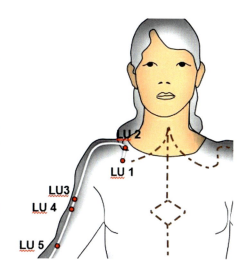

PERICARDIUM 6 - INNER GATE - Calming the flames

Location: This point is three finger widths beyond the wrist on the inside of the forearm in between the two tendons

Session: Using the Grip technique, apply slight pressure with your thumb to the PC 6 point. Channel the flow of Ki into this point. When you feel guided to release, repeat the procedure on the other PC 6 point.

Effects: This point is very effective in calming the spirit and decreases anxiety. May be used when the recipient is indicating agitation from work or family stress situations.

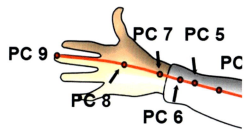

PERICARDIUM 7 - GREAT MOUNT - Protecting the heart

Location: This point is in the middle of the wrist above the palm. It is located in the depression just below the crease of the wrist.

Session: Use the Grip technique to apply slight pressure with your thumb to the PC 7 point. Feel the energy at this point. When you feel guided to release, repeat the procedure on the other PC 7 point.

Effects: Use this point when the recipient is indicating emotional extremes. Highly emotional outbursts may be disruptive to the balance of energy and the consequences manifest as dis-ease. The Pericardium is the Heart's Protector and this is a point that exercises that role.

TRIPLE HEATER 5 - OUTER FRONTIER GATE - Overcoming insecurities

Location: On top of the forearm, two thumb widths beyond the wrist. You will find it in the depression, centred between the bones and tendons.

Session: Using the Grip technique, apply slight pressure with your thumb to the TH 5 point. Consciously direct the flow of Ki into this point. When you feel guided to release, repeat the procedure on the other TH 5 point.

Effects: Use this point to assist the recipient with the ability to overcome timidity and express themselves with confidence.

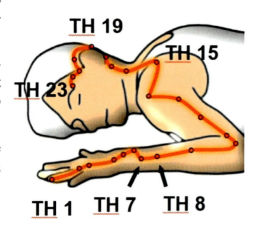

TRIPLE HEATER 17 - WIND SCREEN - Becoming care-free

Location: This point is in the depression behind the earlobe, just below the ear,

Session: Using the Two Finger technique, apply slight pressure with your finger the TH 17 point. You may do both points if the recipient is lying on their back, or one at a time when lying face down. Channel the flow of Ki into this point, as you exhale.

Effects: This point is a very powerful release point for those too concerned about what others think of them. It also assists in letting go of the feelings of shame and guilt.

KIDNEY 3 - SUPREME STREAM - Fearless empowerment

Location: On the inside of the foot, at the midpoint of the depression between the Achilles tendon and the ankle bone.

Session: Cradle the foot in your hand and using the Grip technique, apply pressure with your thumb to the K 3 point. Consciously direct the flow of Ki into this point. When you feel guided to release, repeat the procedure on the other K 3 point.

Effects: This point releases fear and can help to empower a person being able to take a stand. This point is also effective in relieving anxiety and insomnia.

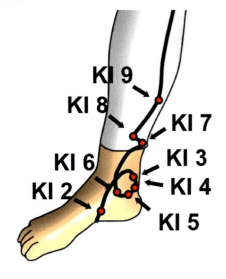

KIDNEY 6 - SHINING SEA - Flowing with grace and ease

Location: On the inside of the foot, in the recess slightly below the front of the ankle bone.

Session: Once again, cradle the foot in your hand and using the Grip technique, apply pressure with your thumb to the K 6 point. Consciously direct the flow of Ki into this point. When complete, repeat the procedure on the other K 6 point.

Effects: This session transmutes the effects that conditioned fear has had on the body and enhances the ability to flow through life with grace and ease. It also increases the recipient's intuitive powers.

LARGE INTESTINE 4 - UNION VALLEY - Inspired living

Location: On top of the hand, at the top of the web between thumb and index finger.

Session: Cradle the recipient's wrist in your hand and using the Grip technique, apply pressure with your thumb to the LI 4 point. Transport the flow of Ki into this point. When you feel guided to release, repeat the procedure on the other hand.

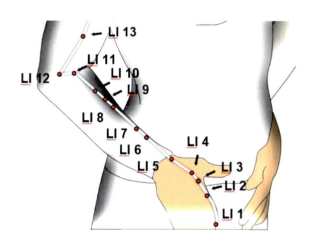

Effects: This "Valley" is also called the Great Eliminator because of its ability to flush out toxic thoughts and habits. Once released the recipient is able to find inspiration and create a life that is more in harmony with their authentic self.

LARGE INTESTINE 11 - CROOKED POND - Freeing the prisoner

Location: On the side of the elbow outside of the arm. You can find it in the depression that is located at the end of the elbow's crease when the arm is bent.

Session: Hold the recipient's wrist in your hand and using the Grip technique, grasp the forearm and apply slight pressure with your thumb to the LI 11 point. Transport the flow of Ki into this point. When you feel guided to release, repeat the procedure on the other arm.

Effects: This point is an important release point. It assists in letting go of what the recipient feels is "justifiable" anger. Although they may feel they should hold onto this anger for what they perceive is a good reason, they are reaping the consequences of the emotion of anger within their body. Balancing the Ki in this meridian at this point allows them the freedom they require to evolve emotionally, mentally and spiritually. It also releases the physical effects that anger has had on their body.

SMALL INTESTINE 5 - YANG VALLEY - Experiencing self-determination

Location: This point is found on the little finger side of the hand. It is in the depression (between the pad and the bone) near the wrist crease, just beyond the wrist bone.

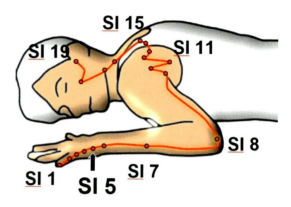

Session: Hold the recipient's hand with one hand and using the Grip technique with the other hand apply slight pressure with your thumb to the SI 5 point. Channel Ki into this point. When you feel guided to release, repeat the procedure on the other arm.

Effects: This point improves clarity, increases the ability to focus, and facilitates discernment.

This session will empower the recipient with better decision-making skills and enable them to write their own script instead of staying in the rut that others have determined for them.

SMALL INTESTINE 19 - PALACE OF HEARING - Listening to your heart

Location: In front of the small projection (called the Tragus) that is in front of the ear canal. This point can be found in the depression that forms on the cheek when the mouth is opened.

Session: Use the Two finger technique and apply slight pressure to the SI 19 point. Direct the flow into this point. When you feel guided to release, repeat the procedure on the other side.

Effects: Balanced energy here will increase intuition and strengthen one's ability to follow their heart. It also facilitates compassion and empathy. This opens the recipient to the heart-felt requirements of those around them.

CONCLUSION

I trust this has been for you, a rewarding and fascinating journey. It certainly has been for me. As with all things we learn in life, Reikiatsu is part of a growth process, and what we do with what we have learned will always be up to us. My hope is that Reikiatsu will be assimilated into your practice and that you will contribute to its evolution by using it to assist others to find balance and harmony in body, mind, and soul.

Currently, there is a worldwide trend to almost epidemic proportions in technological advancement. Social media, artificial intelligence, and electronic communication are truly connecting us all on a global scale. It seems to me, however, that we need to balance this trend with both emotional growth and physical intimacy that are expressed as meaningful, and heart-centred experiences.

Reikiatsu may be thought of as a way to communicate energy through touch and intention. Source energy is what truly connects us all. It is where Unity Consciousness resides. By connecting, in this way, we help to balance the Yin and Yang of our Collective Consciousness.

The world of technology is sometimes seen as bleak and sterile. However, if we are able to mature and open our hearts to our innate relationship with the earth, and all those that share life upon it, we are doing a great service to ourselves and future generations.

Reikiatsu is not the only way, but it is one that provides a wonderful platform for us to connect with ancient oriental wisdom and apply it to our present modern world.

May it bless you and bring you happiness, abundance, balance and joy.

Paul N. Beshara, June 15th, 2017

ABOUT THE AUTHOR

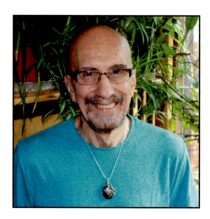

While working as an Addiction Program Director in Ottawa, Ontario, Canada, Paul Beshara began searching for something that would open him energetically to alternative methods of health and well-being. The wonderful flow of Reiki accomplished that for him, and he became a Reiki practitioner in 1993. He later went on to become a Reiki Master in 1998.

Upon furthering his studies in Shiatsu, and Orthotherapy, he left the addictions field in 2000 and opened his own holistic therapy clinic in Winchester, Ontario. Paul also received certification as a Certified Clinical Hypnotherapist, Certified Acu-Hyno Practitioner, Certified Hypnotist, and as a Certified Neuro-linguistic Programming Practitioner.

During these years of holistic practice, he began to combine his understanding of the Meridian System and his Reiki practice and found that he was experiencing significant results.

In 2012, Paul closed his clinic and moved on to become the publisher of Natural Presence Magazine, an Eastern Ontario magazine dedicated to mind, body, and soul.

Now, at the glorious age of 70 and retired, Paul has made the decision to share his perspective on the complementary modalities of Reiki and the Meridian System.

Reikiatsu: The Reiki Practitioner's Guide To Working With The Meridians, is Paul's first book on the union of these two complementary systems.

Made in the USA
Columbia, SC
06 July 2017